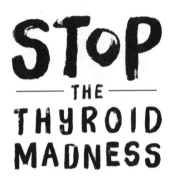

STOP

—— THE ——

THYROID
MADNESS

*A Patient Revolution
Against Decades of
Inferior Thyroid Treatment*

UPDATED REVISION

Janie A. Bowthorpe, M.Ed.

Laughing Grape Publishing, LLC

This book is compiled to provide information and education. Its publication and sale is not intended to replace the relationship with your doctor, medical or pharmaceutical professional and their guidance, and it does not constitute the practice of medicine. Neither the publisher, nor the author, nor any patient mentioned or quoted, nor any of the medical, health or wellness practitioners mentioned, takes responsibility for any consequences from any treatment, procedure, health modifications, actions, or application of any method by any person reading or following the information in this book.

Before undertaking any course of treatment or modification, the author and publisher recommend that you consult with your physician or medical professional regarding any prescription drugs, vitamins, minerals, food supplements or other treatments and therapies that would be beneficial for your particular health problems or dosages that would be best for you.

Every effort has been made to make this book as complete and accurate as possible. However, there may be mistakes, both typographical and in content. Therefore, this book should only be used as a guide, not as the ultimate source of information on thyroid, adrenal and related health issues. Furthermore, this book contains information that is current only up to the printing date.

Library of Congress Cataloging-in Publication Data
Bowthorpe, Janie A
Stop the Thyroid Madness: A Patient Revolution Against
Decades of Inferior Treatment / Janie A. Bowthorpe, M.Ed.
Includes bibliographical references and index.
ISBN 978-0-615-47712-1
1. Hypothyroidism - Popular Works I. Title

LCCN: 2011906208   LOC Classification: RC648-665   Dewey: 616.4/44

Cover design & interior layout by *Olivier Darbonville*

$\mathcal{S}$ending a high five to the many brave thyroid patients all over the world, including those who have...

- autoimmune Hashimoto's
- other forms of thyroiditis
- non-autoimmune hypothyroidism of any cause
- thyroid cancer
- had their thyroid removed
- hypopituitary
- post Graves' hypothyroidism

and who have posted in groups related to Stop the Thyroid Madness (STTM) since 2002 to the present, which enabled me to compile everything YOU have learned and reported, in order to help others.

Whatever you do,
don't look
at the last page
of this book.

D *edicated to "Miserable Mom"–the handle of a gal who posted on a health web site, got a lousy answer from the doctor which only kept her sick, and who was the final impetus for me to start the Stop the Thyroid Madness Revolution with sweet revenge. I hope you find this book.*

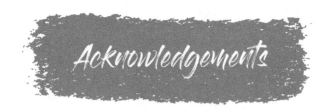
Acknowledgements

Not one inch of this now newly-updated revision would have been possible without the continued throngs of thyroid patients worldwide who gather in social media groups, ask their questions, demand change from their doctors, explore, read, and share it all so we can learn from each other. I was one of those patients early on, and I've worked with and been blessed by countless others.

There are important updates in every single chapter, in many places, small or large (other than my story). There are important updates throughout both adrenal chapters. There are numerous updated URLs. There is updated info about thyroid meds, adrenal meds, additions to the good foods and supplements. There is an improved layout plus formatting changes! Some paragraphs are slimmed down; others revamped. Even to this very day, we continue to learn and fine-tune what we have seen and experienced before, thus why this updated revision was needed!

It all started in 2002 when I created a Yahoo group for all of us. That was before Facebook! Why did I start all this? Because the medical community was simply keeping us sick! And I knew that getting well again had to be based on our collective experiences and wisdom as patients who lived it!

Then came the beginning of the Stop the Thyroid Madness website in late 2005, when I started compiling all we were learning in getting well again. That compiling process continues to this very day as we tweak and refine. Then the growth and expansion of Facebook over the years that birthed the Stop the Thyroid Madness (STTM) Facebook page. And now the STTM books!

This important and life-changing book, totally based on

years of reported patient experiences and observations rather than empty strong opinion, acknowledges all of **you** from 2002 to this very day.

I would be amiss if I didn't mention some great doctors at the beginning of this patient-to-patient movement that deserve recognition for helping us along the way: David Derry, MD; Dr. William McK Jeffries, Barry Durrant Peatfield, LRCP MRCS, John Dommisse, MD; Joseph Mercola, DO; Bruce Rind, MD; Michael Lam, MD; Gina Honeyman DC; John C. Lowe, DC,. And last but not least, the book which was the catalyst for it all by Dr. Broda Barnes: *Hypothyroidism: The Unsuspected Illness.* He knew even in the 1950's that we need NDT and/or T3 in our treatment.

Even today, in spite of the medical profession having a long way to go to get out of their dark age poor understanding, we do see more doctors willing to listen and learn! Progress. But more is needed, as we STILL see information put on the net that is so off, just as we hear bad info from our doctors.

And as always, I have to continually give thanks to my dear husband for his patience when his wife spends innumerable hours on the computer over the years as the owner of many groups, the creator of the huge Stop the Thyroid Madness website (which is always a continual job), a blogger, speaker, coach and author.

There's even now another very important book called *Hashimoto's: Taming the Beast.*

And to my sons who played many roles in helping me be far more informed about the creation of a website and where to look for help on the net in doing so.

Finally, even if this sounds a bit hokey, I'm a cat person And I give deep thanks to the cats I have loved, all through these editions, who in turn gave that love back to ME!

Janie A. Bowthorpe, M. Ed.

*M*ost of what Stop the Thyroid Madness is about is years of worldwide patient repeated reports, strong experiences, and the wisdom gained from all those years of the latter. That is purposeful to avoid the missteps of "strong opinion" or spurious, made up information.

And because continuing experiences and wisdom are part of a dynamic process, Janie Bowthorpe will add any new info (that would pertain to what is written in this book), on this page:

http://stopthethyroidmadness.com/book-updates

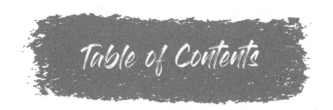

Table of Contents

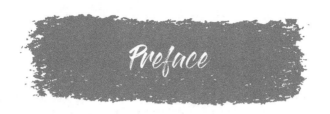

Disgust can have sweet effects. It was around Summer of 2005, and I had been observing a large health web site for a few months. On the thyroid forum, I was seeing certain posters disappear, one by one, to post no more.

Why? I could see the trend. If they dared to mention desiccated thyroid to someone else rather than the T4-only like Synthroid or Levothyroxine praised by the doctor; if they dared to disagree with the doctor that the TSH is a good treatment guide; if they dared to say that the free T3 may be a better lab; they were being kicked off. It was disgusting.

It's also where I first saw the words of a gal who called herself *Miserable Mom*, and to whom this book is dedicated. She described a slew of miserable symptoms, only to be told by the well-meaning but highly misinformed doctor that her two grains of porcine Natural Desiccated Thyroid were adequate and from a thyroid standpoint, there wasn't more to do. I was appalled. She was clearly under-dosed, had been miserable for ten years, and was going to stay so based on that forum advice.

And that very day, out of my anger and disgust, is when the Stop the Thyroid Madness ball started to roll in my mind. If doctors were going to continue to be as *brainless as a block of wood*–leaving patients sick, confused and tired–a different direction had to be taken: patients educating patients, and that information to be taken assertively and confidently into the doctor's office.

This book is not my opinion, my observation, my direction. Its compilation represents the *opinion, observation and direction of hundreds of thousands of patients (if not more) who have struggled together to find answers via numerous internet groups and forums.* I am simply the messenger who named the revolution and compiled the brilliance of what thyroid patients have learned and reported.

I would say that nothing in this book is perfect. But most of what you are going to read is extremely close, and the rest will evolve as this patient revolution continues. We are getting well again!

And again, there are several important updates in every single chapter (other than My Story), whether updated URL's, updated product names, updated treatment details.   There are important updates throughout both adrenal chapters. There is an improved layout plus formatting changes! Some paragraphs are slimmed down; others revamped. Even to this very day, we continue to learn and fine-tune what we have seen and experienced before, thus why this updated revision was needed!

The hope of this book? That you will become *enlightened and empowered* by the hard-earned knowledge and success given in these pages, and carry that information into your doctor's office, *demanding a far better treatment protocol, as well as respect for your own knowledge and inner wisdom.*

And if you don't get regard and attentiveness about your own knowledge and wisdom from one doctor, you will move on... and move on again until you do. We, as patients, will change the blundering thyroid treatment medical monster from the bottom up with our knowledge, our persistence, and our pocketbooks.

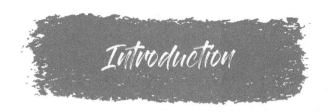
Introduction

*If a thousand old beliefs were ruined
on our march to truth, we must still march on.*

STOPFORD BROOKE

MY STORY

I t wasn't more than several years ago that I was sitting on the front cedar deck of my home gazing at the red hue of the late afternoon clouds…and crying. Granted, I was in a happy marriage with a tall cowboy, and I was awed by the views from my front and back decks. When you have lived in the flatlands of Texas for most of your life, nothing beat what I could see from my house now.

But, my ability to physically live my life was going down the tubes.

Sure, the previous 20 years had been difficult enough, with nearly all of those years on Synthroid and later Levoxyl—both T4-only medications and just like what is called levothyroxine. But I had managed and made the best of it, even if frustrated, limited, and often miserable.

Now, I was seeing an even more debilitating decline for two years. I couldn't be on my feet for more than 30 minutes without extreme tiredness setting in and the soles of my feet hurting as if I was standing on glass shards. If my husband and I attended any event that involved standing, I was now forced to bring a small moveable stool to sit on. It was humiliating.

Even worse, if I dared go beyond my already-limited energy range, I would move into the same bizarre and debilitating physical overreaction I had been living with for two decades.

Just the day before, while sitting and after I had used sandpaper to smooth the edges of a small wood project, I ended up no less exhausted than a marathon runner. My heart pounded violently in my chest. The fatigue was nauseating. I had terrible insomnia that night. And I was disabled the next day. It was very akin to what is called Dysautonomia, an extreme overreaction by one's autonomic nervous system.

When my husband came out and sat by me on that deck, I had to look straight into his eyes with tears in my own and say *"I need your help to apply for Social Security Disability."* I also knew I would become dependent on my husband to even grocery shop. It was a low, low moment.

How it all began

It was 1979. I was pregnant with my second child. And around the 8th month, I began having very strange mental aberrations. I would wake up feeling strangely disconnected from my body, as if my thoughts were far, far away and difficult to express. It was frightening, but it ceased when I gave birth.

But after that birth, I was to begin nine months of hell while nursing my son. I had multiple illnesses that included a minimum of four colds (just as one ended, a new one would begin), a bronchial infection, a flu-like illness and finally viral pneumonia. And two-and-a-half years later, I had a similar scenario while nursing my third son, namely, a succession of viral illnesses followed by bacterial pneumonia and the worst flu I'd ever had months after that.

Finally, the illnesses stopped, but a new frustrating saga was to begin. I was unable to hold my babies or toddlers for very long. My arms felt like dead weights with extreme weakness. I had to continually pass my young children over to my husband.

By the time I was 29 years old and had three healthy young sons, I concluded that my easy arm fatigue and poor stamina was due to being out of shape. I then decided to begin a career as a fitness instructor, receiving top notch certifications from the Aerobic Institute in Dallas. I started my own fitness business in the basement of a church when I was 30 years old, teaching five one-hour classes weekly.

But something quite bizarre was going on after each and every class. Instead of recovering from the workout, my heart rate would stay high, and by 8-9 pm each evening, I would be a basket case of debilitating and profound fatigue. When I went to bed for the evening, my heart would pound in my chest as if I had an internal hammer. I was as weak as if someone took a drinking straw to my body and sucked out all the energy. My fatigue would be so pronounced that I felt nauseous. I would have insomnia for hours, and I would sweat like a pig. The next morning, I felt no better than if I had been run over by an 18-wheeler and smashed against a concrete wall.

Thinking this strange reaction would pass, I prevailed, building my business and creating a fitness newsletter for my clients. But it didn't go away. And I was yawning through any school event I attended for my sons, and suffering.

I made an appointment with our doctor, and via a TSH test, he pronounced me *"borderline hypothyroid"* with a result of 5.2 (which is high!). I was placed on Synthroid, raised to 100 mcg. When my TSH came down into the 2's, I was pronounced adequately treated and would have no more problems! Needless to say, I was thrilled. I loved my new fitness profession and looked forward to building a strong business.

Wrong.

After 2 years of teaching fitness classes, I was forced to give up my beloved career due to my body's continuing bizarre and extremely debilitating reaction to each and every class. I was just plain exhausted to the bone and it was compromising my abilities as a mom, as well.

Nearly two decades of problems

And for the next 17 years, while "adequately treated" on Synthroid and later Levoxyl (T4-only) with a "target TSH"---even with lowering that TSH---I was to go through more periodic hell.

- I was unable to do active outdoor activities with my children without paying a physical price.
- I was unable to spend time shopping or walking with friends due to my lack of stamina.

- I was limited in my abilities on vacations with my family due to my poor stamina and highly extreme reactions to exercise or the sun.
- I was unable to play volleyball on a local neighborhood team due to paralyzing weakness in my arms just 15 minutes into the game.
- I had to choose jobs carefully to avoid long-term standing and movement.
- I had to deal with chronic low-grade depression, even though I was "adequately treated".
- I had to take frequent naps to get by.
- If I tried to do any activity away from home, I was forced to take a day and more off to 'recover' from the debilitating results.

I remember being on vacation with my family, walking across a large field to view old archeological mounds. It was a beautiful and hot sunny day, and the terrain was flat. When we returned to the car an hour later and resumed our driving, my debilitating fatigue from walking and my overreaction to the sun we were in became so profound that I told my husband I needed to be taken to a hospital. I outright felt like death warmed over and couldn't keep my eyes open. We kept driving to our next motel, though, and I collapsed in bed.

I spent thousands upon thousands of dollars trying to find out what was wrong over those years, and amassed a thick stack of lab work, to no avail. I was always "adequately treated" with T4-only medications. I even raised my medications to further lower my "target" TSH into the ones.

Tests, treatments and too many diagnoses

During these 17 years, I drove thousands of miles, saw a broad slew of doctors and was tested and experimented on for every condition imaginable:

- I did tests for hypoglycemia.
- I was a guinea pig for a doctor's hormonal treatment.
- I had a painful muscle biopsy.
- I did the adrenal ACTH Stim test.
- I tried homeopathic remedies.

- I had blood drawn for every hormone problem.
- I did a treadmill test.
- I took beta blockers.
- I wore a heart monitor.
- I did bizarre and painful neurological tests.

I was told I was depressed. I was told I had Chronic Fatigue Syndrome, also known as myalgic encephalomyelitis (ME) in Europe and the UK. I was told I had an unusual "energy metabolism disorder." I was tested for Glycogen Storage Disease. I was told I have a serious but unknown "mitochondria disorder"–a prognosis which would only get worse. And on my own, I saw similarities in my symptoms to Dysautonomia, an overreaction of the autonomic nervous system, and named my condition "post-exercise dysautonomia." But never, ever was there any conclusive diagnosis as to what I had, and 'it was never my thyroid'.

When my hair became thinner and thinner, I was simply told I had alopecia. And like millions of silent patients around, I became a member of the Yaya Hypohood Psychiatrists Club (Chapter 10)—falling for the premise that I MUST have a psychological problem causing all this. What a bunch of hogwash. It was a waste of my money.

The façade of looking normal

And the most remarkable aspect of all the above: I doubt *anyone* who has known me would say I appeared to be anything less than normal. Namely, though all the above occurred just as you read it, I still raised three children, had my own jewelry line, kept up the houses we lived in, made each Christmas special, each birthday memorable, got a Master's Degree, had a private business in counseling, led many continuing education self-help college classes, taught in public school a few years, participated in archaeological digs, and kept exercising by walking. *But I paid horrific and nauseating prices often and privately, and I adapted my life all over the place just to be able to do some of the above.* Many of us are just like this, in our own degree and kind, when on a thyroxine T4-only medication like

Synthroid, Levoxyl or any of numerous levothyroxine brands around world, including Oroxine, Eltroxin and others.

By 2002, my physical fatigue and bodily overreactions became so pronounced that I found myself sitting on that front deck with the beautiful sunset, asking my husband to help me apply for Social Security Disability. It had been a long road, looking healthy and normal in the eyes of friends and acquaintances around me. I have no doubt that anyone who knew me back then would be quite surprised what I was going through. But I was living miserably, typical of an invisible illness. And for all I knew, I now had one foot in the grave.

The beginning of change

But, 2002 was going to be a new beginning. Because I could do nothing else, I became obsessed with research and my computer was smoking. I always think of the five steps of grief as identified by Elizabeth Kübler-Ross: Denial, Anger, Bargaining, Depression, and Acceptance. To my favor, I had never stayed in the "Acceptance" phase very long. I kept fighting against the idea that I was headed for disability.

And though it took a few months, I found patients in a small Yahoo group mentioning a prescription medication called natural desiccated thyroid, their problems with T4-only treatment, and the fallacy of the TSH lab. Whoa! I was like the cartoon character with springs behind my eyes. I found a possible answer! What I was reading seemed to imply that desiccated thyroid, which at that time was the popular brand name of Armour, was changing their lives.

And I proved it. I found a Nurse Practitioner (NP_ over an hour away from me who would help me switch to Armour in July of 2002. Unfortunately, she left me on my starting dose of ¾ grain for nine weeks, which caused a return of my hypo- symptoms. I then moved to another NP who had more understanding of raising your dose. And no kidding... my life began to change 180 degrees!

I first noticed that no longer was I having that bizarre and highly debilitating physical reaction to activity. Gone! Kaput! I had to pinch myself. Was this real? Would it creep back up on me when I wasn't looking? Nope, it didn't. And considering how disabling those reactions to anything physical had been for so long, this in itself was a huge miracle.

As I increased the desiccated thyroid with its direct T3, I saw my hair and skin soften. I now had soft, strokable hair rather than a brillo pad. I also now had a healthy oiliness at my roots rather than a week of dry hair before I had to wash it.

Next, I saw an abatement of my chronic low-grade depression and regained an inner smile.

Then I saw my constipation change, my weak arms and legs become strong, and my painful feet disappear. For the first time in years and years, I could stand for hours and survive!!

And now I could have an active day and NOT have to lie on the couch in front of the evening TV news and fall into a snoozing la-la land. I could come home from an active day and do housework! (A dubious joy but still glad.)

Some improvements took longer than others, such as the return of my once-thick hair, but improve it did! And best of all, I regained my energy and stamina.

By 2003, I was a different person and I loved it. I could stand for long periods of time without an issue. I could exercise without an issue. I could buy groceries without an issue. I could *live*...without an issue.

Was it and has it been a smooth transition to better health and renewed energy? Nope. When I had regained most of the above, I had to figure out twice in a few years that I had low serum iron, which in turn caused me to slide into iron anemia twice with miserable symptoms similar to the worst hypothyroid. So, I had to correct it. I had to give myself far better supplements to meet the new energy demands of my body. I had to correct female hormonal issues possibly brought on by the long years of staying hypothyroid. I had to deal with highly stressed adrenals. I also found myself with low potassium and low magnesium which needed correction. But I got through those boulders on the thyroid yellow brick road.

Until you've been at the bottom of your particular pit, and climbed out, you'll never know what it's like to be human again... to be able to spend hours doing what you love, to hike to places you only wished you could see, to be outside and enjoy the memory, to run a business, to participate in group physical activities, and to just plain *live*. I can now sit on any deck, glancing at the beauty all around me, and then walk down the steps and do whatever I want to do without horrendous consequences!

8 Common experiences we all share

There are unique and individual facets of my story. Some you might identify with; others you might not. *But there are still common factors in my story shared by most any hypothyroid patient around the world. They are:*

1. **Millions of us are put on a T4-only treatment** as if it's the only acceptable treatment out there. And it's not acceptable when we are forced to get the active hormone T3 via conversion alone.
2. **We aren't made aware that there are too many issues which can hinder the conversion of T4** to the active hormone T3. I'll go over those in Chapter 1.
3. **Millions who think they are doing great on T4 have lingering symptoms** of an inadequate treatment and don't put two-and-two together.
4. **Most all of us have, or have had, lab-obsessed doctors who are not paying attention** to our clinical presentations/symptoms of the failure in living for conversion alone to T3.
5. **We are band-aided with medications** to cover lingering symptoms up, or told to see a Psychiatrist/Psychologist
6. **We are all being held hostage to the lousy TSH lab** and the ridiculous "normal" range. It's a pituitary hormone, not a thyroid hormone, and it can look "normal" for years while we get worse and worse!
7. **Doctors fail to go by the free T3 and free T4,** or fail to understand where those frees need to fall in the ranges. We are not the "normal" setting on a washing machine!

8. **We are all left with symptoms of some kind and of some degree as a result of a substandard treatment with T4-only and the TSH**, even if we fail to understand the connection. It too often leads to the misery of too high or too low cortisol levels, inadequate iron levels, inflammation, low B12, low vitamin D, low minerals, mental health issues like depression or excess anxiety, feeling cold, hair loss, dry skin or hair, rising blood pressure, rising cholesterol, aches and pains, poor immune function (especially awful if we have Hashimoto's) and much more.

And on the other side of the coin, just like myself, a growing body of thyroid patients now have the common experience of switching to *a quality prescription natural desiccated thyroid product,* or even treating with both synthetic T4 and synthetic T3. And with either version of treatment which includes direct T3 in it, we find our *optimal dose which puts the free T3 towards the top part of the range and a free T4 midrange. Both. And to get there, we now know that we have to have* **optimal cortisol and iron to succeed with the raises without problems**. And we feel *far* better.

A revolution for better treatment has arisen among patients who are standing up against decades of thyroid treatment which has been inferior, rigid and just plain stupid. I am raising the banner, and I hope you will join with me and the growing body of other thyroid patients around the world who are shouting:

STOP THE THYROID MADNESS!

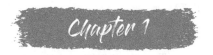

Chapter 1

T4-ONLY TREATMENT GETS A BIG FAT "F"

t's been matter-of-factly going on since the 1960's: a patient is finally given the diagnosis of *hypothyroid* by a doctor, and the prescribed medication is *synthetic levothyroxine sodium*, also simply called *l-thyroxine* or just plain *T4*. Brand names can include *Synthroid, Levoxyl, Levothroid, Eltroxin, Oroxine, Unithroid, generic Levothyroxine, Tirosint and others.*

We thought we were adequately and competently treated with our thyroid medications. Why? Because our doctors told us we were; because the TSH lab said we were; because doctors know what's right for us; because there were 'some' improvements. We've dutifully picked up our prescriptions at our local pharmacy and mindlessly popped our single pill each and every morning. We've felt secure in our treatment and maintained faith in our doctor.

But it's all been blunderingly and scandalously wrong.

How it has happened

From the time they were first created in pill form, T4 medications have been thrust upon the worldwide market and towards hundreds of millions of googly-eyed and trusting hypothyroid or Hashimoto's patients worldwide like a bulldog. It's been used in studies and promoted in medical journals. It's been underscored in pharmaceutical pow-wows and stamped with approval in continuing education conferences. Your friendly-suited pharmaceutical rep has carried it to innumerous doctors' offices with free samples and tasty incentives over the years. Do an internet search of any brand of T4 and you'll get a vast slew of results. Billions of dollars have been invested in its promotion, salability and information machine.

You'll even see Synthroid advertised in 2015 as the number one 'brand name drug' as far as the amount of prescriptions written by physicians.

And what a braggadocios advertising waste of our attention!

In spite of some reported improvements, behind all pharmaceutical promotions are those millions of us as thyroid patients who have been left under-treated/poorly treated with T4-only...sooner or later. It's a treatment which has diminished, to one awful degree or another, our quality of life.

The failure of T4-only in my own family

Many years before I was born, when she was around 20 years old, my mother developed hyperthyroid before she became hypothyroid, aka Graves' disease.

A hyperthyroid condition refers to an over-active thyroid, causing it to produce an overabundance of thyroid hormones. She became as thin as a bean pole. And the recommended solution was surgery to remove most of her thyroid, leaving a very small portion. This is my mother around age 20, thin with Graves'.

Years later, after she married and had two young children, her hyperthyroidism redeveloped complete with bulging eyes–a common symptom. (*And as a young child, I thought my mother was turning into a large insect.*) This time, they used radioactive iodine[1] treatment (RAI) to kill off the small remaining part of her thyroid to prevent further damage from the hyper state.

And sometime after the RAI, when sluggishness of hypothyroidism was starting to appear, she was put on levothyroxine sodium, also called l-thyroxine or simply T4... a *"new and modern"* hypothyroid treatment with the brand name of Synthroid. T4, the thyroid storage hormone, is the most abundant hormone produced by the thyroid. Its main function is to convert to the active and life-giving hormone T3. It was meant to be a story with a happy ending.

But it turned into a Synthroid nightmare

[1] http://stopthethyroidmadness.com/rai

As time progressed, she developed chronic and debilitating depression and became an invisible member of the YaYa Hypohood Psychiatrist Club with chronic depression. (Chapter 10). She spent countless hours in counseling, either with the professionals recommended by her doctor or with a qualified minister of her church.

By the time I was ten, her depression was so severe that she submitted herself to Electric Shock Therapy (EST), a barbaric procedure which was thought to alter the brain and improve depression. I'll never forget my father coming into my room on the day she was coming back home, and saying *"Mama will not remember where the sewing basket is"*.

Never was a treatment more futile. Not only did it dull her sharp intelligence, she remained depressed and was put on antidepressants for the rest of her life—the latter which made her chronically and emotionally apathetic about what was going on around her, or how she made people feel.

Over the years while on T4, she gained weight and dieting produce few results. She had to nap daily. She required long hours to sleep. She never had the stamina of her friends. She couldn't stand on her feet long. She had to forgo certain activities. Her hair was dry. She developed high cholesterol later in life, and a balloon procedure on her heart.

Though she lived until she was 83 with some memorable times, her life was always one of compromise. And though no one figured it out at the time, and my mother went to her grave without knowing...all the above were due to her T4-only treatment: her depression, her weight gain, her poor stamina, her heart issues and high cholesterol, the compromises of her activities... all of it. It was to be a treatment which leaves millions of us hypothyroid to one degree or another.

Common to millions on a T4-only treatment

The details and severity may be different, but the outcome is the same: a life that forever deals with the effect of inadequate T4-only treatment...some less severe, some more severe. And almost as bad are the countless times we noticed a symptom here and there, complained to our doctor, only to be told it's something else, and here's another pill to relieve it. Or the inevitable and insulting *"You need to eat less and exercise more"* if you are in the majority about gaining weight on T4-only, or having a terrible time trying to lose weight.

"But I feel fine!" you may exclaim as you read this.

And I believe you. Some T4 users really do feel better than others. But I also know three facts from communicating with or observing the comments of hundreds of thousands of T4-only thyroid patients over the years:

1. *No matter how fine you feel, you can be living with symptoms related to an inadequate treatment, and you're not putting two-and-two together.*
2. *Feeling fine is subjective, and T4-only treated thyroid patients lower their standards of what "fine" is. That is unfortunately very common.*
3. *The body is not meant to live on a storage hormone alone, and the longer you stay on T4, the more things happen to negatively affect the conversion to T3.*

T4 is simply that—*a storage hormone.* And it has to be converted to T3, the active thyroid hormone, before you can get benefit. T4 is tucked away into the cells of your liver for conversion—the main place it converts. It also happens in your brain, gut, skeletal muscle, heart, and your thyroid gland itself. It's stored away just as you place that jar of grandma's jam in the pantry for another time.

Yet a healthy thyroid makes not just the storage T4, but also direct T3—it doesn't force you to live for conversion of T4 to T3 alone.

Lingering symptoms on T4-only treatment

When it was becoming clear that desiccated thyroid, with its T4, T3, T2, T1 and calcitonin, was changing lives, I asked a large body of thyroid patients what symptoms they had while they were on synthetic T4 medications like Synthroid, Levothyroxine, Eltroxin, etc. The resulting list was staggering.

The list is not only profound, but if you really think about the implications, it's disgusting. It's not only a long tally of symptoms experienced by patients while on thyroxine treatment, *but nearly all of them are also untreated hypothyroid symptoms*! In other words, the symptoms reveal that your levothyroxine T4-only treatment leaves you hypothyroid in your own degree and kind. A second ironic qualification was this: *to* ONLY *list symptoms they had while on a T4-only treatment which have now been highly improved or eradicated since being on desiccated thyroid.* Yes, these symptoms had all been lessened, improved or removed when these patients had switched to desiccated thyroid (even adding T3 to their T4) and dosed according to the elimination of symptoms, besides getting their free T4 and free T3 optimal. We'll cover desiccated thyroid in the next chapter.

Lingering Symptoms While on T4-only Medications

Less stamina than others	Carpal tunnel symptoms
Less energy than others	No appetite
Deep exhaustion	Inability to concentrate
Long recovery period	Anxiety
Bad reaction to exercise	Heart Fluid retention
Frequent napping	Heart Palpitations
Inability to hold children	Fast heartrate
Arms feeling heavy	Irregular heartbeat
Chronic low-grade depression	Swollen legs that prevent walking
Chronic severe depression	High Blood Pressure
The need for anti-depressants	Low Blood Pressure
Suicidal thoughts	Low body temperature
Often feeling cold	Tightness in throat; sore throat
Cold hands, feet	Swollen lymph glands
High cholesterol	Hard little round stools
Rising cholesterol	No bowel movements daily
Being on statins	No or thinning eyebrows
Colitis	Dry hair
Irritable bowel syndrome	Dry skin
Constipation	Cracked heels
Inability to eat in the mornings	Ridged fingernails
Joint pain	Hair loss

White new hair growth
Hair breakage
Nodding off
Afternoon naps
Sleep Apnea
Air Hunger
Inner Ear problems
Varicose Veins
Easy weight gain
Inability to lose
Relationship problems
Low sex drive
Crabby or moody
Sad
PMS
Heavy period
Failure to ovulate and/or
  constant bleeding
Problems getting pregnant
Miscarriages
Low iron
Low B12
Low Vitamin D
Aching bones/muscles
Swelling
Puffy ankles or wrists
Osteoporosis
Osteopenia
Bumps on legs

Poor skin quality
Hives
Exhaustion in every dimension
Slowing to a snail's pace
Illegible handwriting
Internal itching of ears
Weak fingernails
Ringing in ears
Foggy thinking/brain fog
Confusion
Forgetfulness
Inability to work full time
Allergies worsening
A cold rear end
Cold knees
Painful bladder
Dysphagia Nerve Damage
Pneumonia
Easy sicknesses
Slow recovery from illness
Worsening PTSD (post-traumatic
  stress disorder)
Overactive Autonomic Nervous
  System (Dysautonomia)
Low aldosterone
Rosacea
Overreaction to cold medications

The history of T4 use

At this point, you may be asking *"If T4-only medication is so inadequate for so many, why did it come into existence anyway?"*

Its history starts around 1914 when the thyroid hormone T4 was first isolated from the rest of the thyroid by a biochemist named *Edward C. Kendall,* which was quite an accomplishment. In association with the University of Minnesota, he was the Head of the Biochemistry Section in the Graduate School of the Mayo Foundation. You can find biographical information on Kendall on the *www.nobelprize.org/* website, and you'll note that in 1950, he received a Nobel Prize for discovering the activity of cortisone. His work as to the isolation of T4 was reported in the *Journal of Biological Chemistry* (JBC), and reveals that the isolation came from 6500 pounds of hog thyroid glands.

Twelve years later, in 1926-27, British chemists *Charles Harrington* and *George Barger* were the first to produce and use synthetic thyroxine T4, and the New York Times reported that fact in the Dec. 12, 1927 issue, titling the article *Britons discover synthetic thyroxin* by T. R. Ybarra. Both also wrote the 1927 book *Chemistry of Thyroxine–Constitution and Synthesis of Thyroxin.*

The first promising experiments with thyroxine

Thyroxine was originally used on two patients, with the first being a 61-year-old housewife named Mrs. A.S., who had success with previous hospital use of thyroid extract (older name for what we now call desiccated thyroid).

Observations of Mrs. A.S. included that she was mentally dull, overweight, swollen, and her face appeared harsh and dry. She was given thyroxine T4 intravenously, and they noted changes. She was "much brighter and more cheerful, her swellings were diminishing, and wrinkling was obvious on the backs of the hands and under the eyes." When they removed the treatment, they saw that her skin became harsh once again, and her basal metabolic rate declined.

The second case was a 35-year-old housewife, Mrs. M.M., who was diagnosed myxedema (older term for hypothyroid) in 1920, and who had not taken her thyroid extract (older term of desiccated thyroid).

When admitted to the hospital in 1926, Mrs. M.M. had a lack of energy and noticeable bodily swellings. After three intravenous injections of synthetic thyroxine, they noted that the thyroxine raised her basal metabolic rate, with a rise in her temperature and pulse. Additionally, she lost weight due to a "great loss of fluid from the system."

Both cases of Mrs. A.S. and Mrs. M.M. revealed that the use of T4 had positive results. But thyroxine never became a worthy treatment. Why? Because relying on an intravenous treatment was not practical. And thyroxine was known to have instability in the presence of light and air. Additionally, desiccated thyroid was working well during that time anyway.

The fact that desiccated thyroid was successful (and remained so for many decades), and synthetic T4 was used intravenously and unstable, should have ended the T4 experiment.

But T4-only as a thyroid treatment was to return to the commercial and public eye thirty-five years later. The late 1950's and early 60's both were a time when pharmaceutical companies started to heavily market and mass-produce their products with $$ signs in their eyes. Additionally, it was a time when false and negative claims were made against desiccated thyroid in several medical articles and journals. It was later identified as a hoax, but the damage was done.

By 1955, Knoll Pharmaceuticals of Germany developed the ever well-known Synthroid, a thyroxine now in tablet form. Dr. David Derry, a noted physician in Canada who graduated from medical school in 1962, stated to me in an email that he noticed a strong swing towards thyroxine treatment by 1963.

A faulty assumption

Today, looking back at the early positive results with thyroxine of Mrs. A.S. and Mrs. M.M, and reading numerous studies and articles about the efficacy of thyroxine use, one might come to a knee-jerk conclusion that levothyroxine sodium, aka T4 or thyroxine, is and has always been a good product in the treatment of hypothyroid. Why else would my doctor prescribe it? Why else would there be hundreds of millions on these medications? Even the Synthroid website states:

> *Synthroid offers safe and effective treatment to patients like you every day. Your thyroid medication is carefully prescribed by your doctor to achieve a delicate balance of thyroid hormone in your body. (Not)*

Additionally, you will find patients who state they are pleased with their T4-only treatment and the alleviation of some symptoms. You, the reader, may feel this way.

Thud

Yet, a pertinent and reflective question remains: how much relief are you really getting from a T4-only treatment? Is 20% enough? 50%? 70%? What if there's no noticeable relief? Because the same conclusion is found in the experience of millions owho find out the truth: *T4-only thyroxine treatment has a negative pattern of improvement and outcome in most thyroid patients in some degree and kind, sooner or later, as shown in the compiled list of continuing symptoms on page 6.*

In other words, in contrast to whatever improvements from a T4-only treatment that can be documented in journals, implied in research, stated on websites, or expressed by patients, the worldwide array of negative results, sooner or later is so widespread that most of can conclude *without a shadow of a doubt*: thyroxine treatment is overall a miserable failure!

In fact, my way of explaining it is this:

> *T4-only medication treatment does the job*
> *to the same degree that an elevator which only rises*
> *to the fifth floor of a 50-story building "does the job."*

Now, a gel form of T4 called Tirosint is a good example of a T4 that can give better conversion results than other versions of T4, as reported by patients. But there are still too many reasons that forcing your body to live for conversion alone can backfire: infections, inflammation, fasting, chronic emotional stress, intense exercise, high heavy metals, liver problems, eating too many goitrogens, leaky gut, low mineral levels, beta blockers, low iron, inflammation, activation of certain mutations, chemo, radiation, cortisol problems.....even aging! Any of the latter can make the conversion backfire! A healthy thyroid, just like a healthy treatment, doesn't force you to live for conversion alone.

Why has T4-only treatment been a huge failure for so many, sooner or later?

Because the human body is not, and never was, meant to

live on a storage hormone alone. You are not meant to live on water alone. You are not meant to live on food alone. You are not meant to live on T4 alone. Instead, your body is meant to optimally live on the entire complement of what your thyroid produces: T4, T3, T2, T1 and calcitonin.

As a result, T4-only treatment has earned an F on the report card of thyroid treatment for far too many. Millions of patients across the world are making it clear that they continue to have lingering symptoms of hypothyroidism, whether perceived to be mild or severe, while on a T4-only treatment...sooner or later.

We don't need research papers, double-blind studies, medical articles, or glowing words in a pharmaceutical handout to tell us that T4-*only, thyroxine medications have near completely failed millions of us sooner...or later...and their use has simply lined the pockets of their makers. There are simply too many situations which can negatively affect that conversion, as explained on the previous page. We need direct T3!*

T4-ONLY TIDBITS

* Have no thyroid? Been put on T4? You all the more need to have T3 in your treatment. Next chapter...

* Humorously stated a few years ago by an insightful patient: "I have found a couple of uses for a bottle of Synthroid: 1) Doorstop 2) Prop for an old DSL modem (so it won't overheat). However, I do not recommend it to be taken internally all by itself. Ever."

* The evidence is strong among thyroid patients: many cases of "fibromyalgia" or "chronic fatigue syndrome" appear on T4-only meds, and go away when optimally treated on desiccated thyroid.[2]

---

[2] http://stopthethyroidmadness.com/fibromyalgia

Chapter 2

SO WHAT DO PIGS HAVE TO DO WITH IT?

I've a right to think," said Alice sharply, for she was beginning to feel a little worried "Just about as much right," said the Duchess, "as pigs have to fly...
ALICE IN WONDERLAND BY LEWIS CARROLL

"**O**h sure. I'm going to have more energy when pigs fly." Yup, that's exactly the sarcastic idiom I would have used if once upon a time, when I was on Synthroid and later Levoxyl, someone had predicted that I was going to have more energy thanks to a pig.

A pig? Nope, I couldn't see a pig helping me. And I had spent too many years of living with constant compromises and miseries in my energy levels, even while a slew of doctors stated it was not my thyroid since I was *"adequately treated"* and my TSH was *"normal."*

But sometimes you just have to eat your bacon. Because lo and behold, not only did the pigs fly, they soared after I had switched from a T4-only medication to a porcine thyroid product, once known as thyroid extract, but now more commonly called *natural desiccated thyroid (NDT)*.

More than a century of desiccated thyroid use

If your ancestors had an identifiable thyroid problem, there's a good chance they were treated with desiccated thyroid.

Desiccated thyroid was to see its medical debut in the late 1800's. And if you put recent dates together, that means hypothyroid patients were using this product successfully for more than five decades before the pharmaceutical T4/levothyroxine money-eyed assault in the late 1950's and early 1960's.

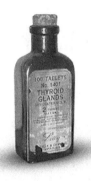

In the early days, desiccated thyroid was either from pigs or sheep. I own a very early bottle of Armour desiccated thyroid, still with the product inside and sealed with a cork. And on the vintage browned label, it states THYROIDS DESICCATED and defines the powder within as fresh thyroid gland of the sheeps [sic]. Today, desiccated thyroid by prescription, also called natural desiccated thyroid, or thyroid extract in older literature, is almost exclusively comprised of whole porcine thyroid glands. Perhaps pigs were ultimately chosen because their tissue can be nicely compatible with our own. That's why pig heart valves are often used in humans who need replacements.

Desiccated refers to the fact that the approved and inspected pig thyroid is frozen, minced, dried and milled into a fine powder. Several batches are combined to create a consistent lot of the full strength porcine thyroid powder. Testing is then done to make sure it meets the established specifications.

There are a few over-the-counter desiccated thyroid products made from grass-fed bovine from New Zealand or Argentina. They have been well received by patients when doctors refuse to prescribe NDT, or keep patients' hostage to the TSH. We occasionally see weaker batches here or there. The goals are the same—to be optimal. For prescription porcine, and if your religious beliefs or vegetarian stance create concern about the use of pork, see Addendum B.

T4-only vs desiccated thyroid meds

Unlike synthetic T4-only medications like Synthroid, Levothyroxine, Eltroxin, Oroxine and others, natural desiccated thyroid (NDT) is just that—natural and not a manmade synthetic. There's nothing wrong with the synthetic versions as being "synthetic", but many patients like that fact that NDT is natural. *[handwritten annotations]*

Even more important to many patients, NDT provides the exact same hormones that your own thyroid would be giving you if healthy. In other words, not just T4, the storage hormone, but also direct T3, as well as T2, T1 and calcitonin. *[handwritten annotation]*

Prescription NDT is measured according to specific amounts of T4 and T3 in one grain–38 mcg T4 and 9 mcg T3 in most brands, and only slightly different amounts in others. It's also stated to be 80% T4 and 20% T3, or the ratio is 4.22 parts of T4 to one part of T3[3]. In most cases, one grain equals 60 mg.

Rumor occasionally goes through the mill that desiccated thyroid is nothing more than T4 and T3, especially since the other thyroid hormones aren't mentioned in descriptions or product paper insert. But pharmaceuticals will assure you that T2, T1 and calcitonin are simply not measured and are there.

> *When describing the T4 and T3 in desiccated thyroid, pharmaceuticals use the same terms as for synthetic versions, aka Liothyronine (T3), and either tetraiodothyronine or levothyroxine (T4). But they are natural versions.*

Most pharmaceuticals press the desiccated thyroid powder into a tablet. Various dosage strengths have included: ¼, ½, 1, 2, 3, 4 and/or 5 grain tablets *depending on the pharmaceutical distributor*. With most, one grain equals 60 mg; others are 65 mg.

Most all desiccated thyroid powders used in the prescribed thyroid medications are labeled Thyroid USP, meaning they meet the high quality and strict standards of the United States Pharmacopeia (USP[4]). The USP is an independent, science- based public health organization. Simply put, they set the standards for what would constitute a good quality medication. You can view their website here: *www.usp.org/about/*.

---

[3] https://www.ncbi.nlm.nih.gov/pubmed/23072197

[4] www.usp.org/

> *By the way, next time your doctor claims that desiccated*
> *thyroid is unstable or unreliable, remind them that strict*
> *USP standards are followed by the makers of prescription*
> *desiccated thyroid, i.e. unstable and unreliable are **not** in*
> *the dictionary of a USP standardized product.*

Examples of brand names / kinds for commercially available prescription desiccated thyroid include[3]:

NP Thyroid *by Acella Pharmaceuticals LLC*
WP Thyroid *by RLC Labs®*
Naturethroid by *RLC Labs®*
Compounded Thyroid USP (often T4/T3 instead) *in the US*
Thyroid *by Erfa Canada 2012 Inc*
Compounded desiccated thyroid in Australia
Thyreogland in Germany
Thyreoidum in Denmark

Note: At any time you are reading this, new brands often come out;
pharmaceutical ownership can change. The latter versions of NDT are
common at the time of this writing.

Acella's version of natural desiccated thyroid, which they named NP Thyroid, appeared on the market in late 2010. Patient reports were excellent, comparing it to the way the older Armour used to be.

The US brand name Armour by Forest Laboratories LLC is the oldest on the market and was the most well-known. It was reformulated in 2009 with a flip-flop in the amount of dextrose and cellulose—dextrose going low and cellulose going high. Patients complained. In 2014, it became the property of the pharmaceutical Activas, and Forest Laboratories was also bought out by 2014. Armour became higher priced and seemed different now to patients. Activas also acquired Allergan, Inc pharmaceutical, and adopted the name Allergan. *(Classic pharmaceutical example of acquisitions and mergers!)*

Naturethroid and WP Thyroid are distributed by RLC Labs (formerly Western Research Labs). The company has been around since the 1930's--an early pharmaceutical for natural desiccated thyroid. In 2017, production ceased for both with RLC stating it was due to a machinery change. When they began to return in 2018, certain patients who got back on the "new" Naturethroid reported return of their hypothyroid symptoms quickly or within several weeks. There seemed to be less complaints about WP once it returned.

Some thyroid patients have used two different desiccated thyroid products from Thailand: Thyroid-S or Thiroyd, both with excellent results and comparable in results to prescription US brands. There are unfortunately many fillers--see page 204. Sriprasit Pharma Co. Ltd. in Thailand, which makes a form for their desiccated thyroid called Thyroid-S, state they also use the same Thyroid USP standard desiccated powder.

Canada's version made by Erfa is simply called Thyroid. One grain at 65 mg contains 35 mcg of T4 and 8 mcg of T3 (as compared to 38/9 in US brands). Erfa's Thyroid retains the ability to be done sublingually, which has met approval by patients. There have been some complaints that it's less effective than it used to be.

Australia's and New Zealand's desiccated thyroid is usually compounded by local pharmacists. Denmark's desiccated thyroid is called Thyreoidum, and Germany has one called Thyreogland. Australian compounding pharmacies use the same Thyroid USP standards desiccated powder.

Five components of desiccated thyroid

Desiccated thyroid contains the same five well-known hormonal components as your own thyroid, all made from iodine, and mostly protein bound. When not bound, they are free. They are:

T4 *(also called l-thyroxine, levothyroxine, or thyroxine)* is the 4-iodine-molecule storage hormone of the thyroid. It's sometimes called the primary hormone, since approximately 80-93% (depending on what you read) of what your thyroid produces is T4. T4's main function is to convert to the active hormone T3 as your body needs it beyond the T3 given directly by a healthy thyroid. About 40% of T4 converts to T3 and the rest goes to mostly Reverse T3 (RT3) as a way to remove unneeded T4. T4 also plays a role in brain formation, as well as brain function. Most T4 is bound by transport proteins; a small amount is "free", i.e. unbound and usable. T4 is meant to cross the cell membranes from your blood.

T3 (also called triiodothyronine) is the 3-iodine-molecule "active hormone" of the thyroid, and is approximately 7-20% of the total direct production by a healthy thyroid. It has the greatest effect on your body's energy level and overall health and well-being. T3 makes its appearance when T4 loses one of its molecules to become T3 – a peripheral (away from the thyroid gland) conversion of T4 to T3. But it's also made directly. It can be four to ten times more active than thyroxine T4. Most T3 is bound by transport proteins: a small amount is "free", i.e. unbound and usable. T3 is meant to cross the cell membranes from your blood[5].

T2 (also called diiadothyronine) is the 2-iodine-molecule hormone which may play a role in the production of the deiodinase enzyme that helps convert T4 into T3. It also appears to have some effect on metabolism, thus playing a role in burning body fat. T2 can be associate with one's mitochondria.

T1 (also called monoiodothyronine or just amine) is a thyroid hormone which may play a role in keeping thyroid function in check and influencing the heart.

T0 is mentioned in some literature as a fifth thyroid hormone. But the information is minimal. If it exists, it may play the same role as T1, or it's inert.

Calcitonin, which is primarily secreted by your thyroid, responds to too-high levels of calcium in the blood. It inhibits the release of more calcium from your bones to the blood, and can play a good role in the prevention or reversal of osteoporosis, as has been experienced by several patients who switched to desiccated thyroid and dosed high enough to alleviate symptoms.

The first documented use of desiccated thyroid

The first successful, medically documented use of desiccated thyroid (then called thyroid extract, or glandular extract) occurred in 1891 with a 46-year-old woman named Mrs. S. It was later documented in the March 1920 *British Medical Journal* by George R. Murray, MD. Murray is stated to be the

---

[5] https://www.ncbi.nlm.nih.gov/pmc/articles/PMC4699302/

first doctor to use animal extractions to treat hypothyroidism (and good for him!) Thyroid Extract at that time was from sheep, but eventually switched to porcine.

When Mrs. S was in her early 40's, family members noted that her speech and actions were slow, and Mrs. S found housework to be difficult. Her physical features also became enlarged, probably due to water retention. Her physicians noted that she had no interest in seeing strangers, and she was sensitive to cold weather. Her body temperature was always low, varying between 95.6 and 97.2, with a pulse between 60-70. She had little facial expression, dry skin, fine and thin hair. Her movements were noted as slow and labored, as was her speech and memory. Her periods had also ceased.

Physicians of that day diagnosed her with an advanced case of hypothyroid, which was then called Myxedema. For a short while was also called Gull's Disease, named after Sir William W. Gull, MD, who in 1874 published his observations in five women suffering from hypothyroidism[6].

It was decided to inject her with thyroid extract, and within three months, great change was noted. Her bodily swellings were gone, and her face had greatly improved in its appearance, as well as expressions. She now spoke more rapidly, answered questions with greater ease, and her memory improved. She was now walking the neighborhood again, and could once more do housework with ease. She was less sensitive to the cold. Her menstruation improved. And her temperatures rose.

Mrs. S was later switched to oral administration (which may have been fried sheep thyroid gland—sounds tasty, don't you think? Gulp.) and by 1918, she was given dry thyroid extract in a tablet form. She maintained her better health for 28 years until she died in 1919. It was documented that she consumed over nine pints of the liquid thyroid extract, which was estimated to come from 870 sheep!

Subsequently, for several decades, patients with Myxoedema (hypothyroid) were treated successfully with porcine thyroid extract (desiccated thyroid or natural thyroid). The porcine may have been chosen because allergic reactions are rare.

---

[6] https://www.optimox.com/iodine-study-15

Medical books and the mention of desiccated thyroid

By the time the 1941 *Goodman and Gilman's Pharmacological Basis of Therapeutics* came out, both thyroxine (Thyroxin, U.S.P.) and dried thyroid gland (Thyroid, U.S.P.) were mentioned, but *dried thyroid gland was called the preferred method of treatment.* Tah-dahhh. Dried thyroid gland was measured according to its iodine content (whereas now, it's measured according to its T4 and T3 content). From the 1951 book called *Modern Medical Counselor* comes the following recommendation on how to treat Myxoedema, which shows desiccated thyroid was still the successful treatment of choice:

Some convenient preparation made from the whole thyroid gland substance is the rational remedy for myxedema. It brings remarkable improvement. The patient feels better, thinks more clearly and looks better. There is likely to be considerable reduction in excess weight[7].

In the 1970, 4th edition of the classic *Pharmacological Basis of Therapeutics* by Goodman and Gilman, desiccated thyroid was still described positively:

Thyroid USP is a highly satisfactory preparation for clinical use. Its continued popularity does not derive merely from a reactionary attitude, although at first sight the preparation might seem to be crude, old-fashioned, and poorly standardized. It is evidently uniformly well absorbed unless it has an enteric coating, and the potency is sufficiently standard that variation cannot be detected clinically if the official preparation is prescribed[8].

An event occurred around 1963 which caused a turnaround in the popularity of desiccated porcine thyroid and the unfortunate swing towards synthetic levothyroxine, T4-only treatment. The same 1970 4th edition of *Pharmacological Basis of Therapeutics* gave the following clue as to what occurred:

---

[7] Page 508

[8] Page 1479

"A few years ago, a large batch of material came into the hands of a number of distributors in the United States and Europe and, although of proper iodine content, it later proved not be thyroid at all. This episode gave thyroid a bad name because several publications about the unreliability of thyroid appeared before the hoax was uncovered[9]."

And it appears physicians from that time on fell for the hoax and the subsequent negative articles without a blink of an eye. Over time, nearly all patients were switched to the highly-touted thyroxine T4-only medications. Newly diagnosed patients were also started on thyroxine. By making this mass change in the way hypothyroid patients were treated, the tragic and far reaching supposition was made that T4 would convert to adequate levels of T3. Not.

Of course, though its speculation, some patients wonder how much the Knoll Pharmaceutical Company, which first tableted Synthroid in 1955 as levothyroxine sodium, played a part in promoting the switch, as well, via strategic and successful promotion. But that successful promotion of T4 since the 1960's has also resulted in decades of unsuccessful treatment of millions of hypothyroid patients.

Old timers who used to be on desiccated thyroid, and who were switched to levothyroxine, state they saw the return of old hypothyroid symptoms but didn't know it was the result of the new medication. They put their blind faith in their doctors. *And what a price we have paid!*

Too many doctors to this day seem to be mindless cattle in the chutes of their pharmaceutically-financed, medical school training, appearing to have no memory or knowledge of the success of desiccated thyroid. No less is the influence of the commission-paid pharmaceutical rep who enters each and every office in his or her nicest suit, brightest teeth, and friendliest

---

[9] Page 1479

smile in order to sell each doctor on the latest drug.

And yet, if certain hypothyroid symptoms persist, what doctor doesn't pull out his handy-dandy prescription pad, or pull that sample off the shelf in order to treat the subsequent undertreated hypothyroid symptoms, such as chronic low-grade depression, rising cholesterol, anxiety, mental health issues like depression or bi-polar, hair loss (alopecia), digestive issues, low B12, low Vitamin D...and so many more symptoms of undertreated, poorly treated hypothyroid. In other words, the body is not meant to live on the conversion of T4 to T3 alone.

The momentum of change by thyroid patients

Though it took nearly five decades of T4-only inadequacies for patients to get wise and dare to question their treatment, the step back to desiccated thyroid seemed to start around the turn of the millennium. Thyroid patient Mary Shomon started her Yahoo Thyroid group in 1999, and mention of Armour desiccated thyroid shows up soon after. The Yahoo Natural Thyroid Hormone Users group started in 2002 by the author of this book as a patient group more focused on desiccated natural thyroid and with more reactionary stance against poor treatment. Several other smaller yet active patient thyroid groups popped up around the same time.

On a humorous note, the 2006 edition of *Goodman & Gilman's Pharmacological Basis of Therapeutics* erroneously yet seriously states:

> *Desiccated thyroid preparations, derived from whole animal glands, contain both thyroxine and triiodothyronine and have highly variable biologic activity, making these preparations less desirable.*

Highly variable biologic activity and less desirable? Patient experience begs to differ.

From this you come to realize that even the "bible of pharmacology" doesn't have it right. As stated above, FDA-approved, prescription desiccated thyroid is made according to the official standards and specifications for consistency of the United States Pharmacopeia (USP).

Additionally, not a patient on desiccated preparations would state that their results are less desirable, especially considering this treatment gives you the same hormones as your own thyroid would have been giving you when healthy.

Patients soar on desiccated thyroid when they dose by the elimination of symptoms, first and foremost, in the presence of adequate cortisol, whether from healthy adrenals or supplementation, and when any other issues are discovered and corrected such as low iron and more. *The proof is in their experience!* So, who are the doctors listening to: the words in a pharmacological textbook...or patients?

The 21st century worldwide patient revolution makes it clear: T4-only treatment leaves patients with lingering symptoms, sooner or later, and a switch to desiccated thyroid brings better results, plus the elimination of ever-present symptoms of an inferior treatment.

DESICCATED THYROID TIDBITS

* Desiccated thyroid has been around over 120 years. That says a lot!

* If you are unable to stand the taste of desiccated thyroid and it needs to be chewed up or done sublingually before swallowing, add your choice of a sweetener.

* It's stated that one grain of NDT, because of the conversion of T4 to T3 along with the direct T3, is equal in effect to 25 mcg of T3. Good to know if you use T4 and T3.

* Remarkably, there are patient reports of atrial fibrillation (A-Fib) which completely reverse thanks to the careful use of natural desiccated thyroid or T3. Work with your doctor.

Chapter 3

WHAT THYROID PATIENTS HAVE LEARNED: THE BIBLE OF OUR EXPERIENCES

*No two minds ever come together without, thereby,
creating a third, invisible, intangible force which may
be likened to a third mind.*
NAPOLEON HILL

A t the dawn of the 21st century, when a growing body of thyroid patients began to switch from *T4-only medications* like Synthroid and Levothyroxine, to *natural desiccated thyroid*, they and their doctors also began to tread new ground. It has been a journey seeking a thyroid treatment bliss, but it hasn't been without ruts in the road. It was a road less traveled.

And because the journey had been new, we as patients had to learn by the seat of our pants. Granted, there were a small handful of insightful doctors and medical professionals in literature that helped us along the way–Peatfield, Derry, Jeffries, Brownfield, Lowe, Dommisse, Rind, to name a few in the early stages of our understanding. But overall, we've had to blaze new trails when the vast majority of our personal doctors either weren't knowledgeable enough, open-minded enough, or cared enough about desiccated thyroid or T3.

So, we were modern pioneers, inspired by the path of hypothyroid patients long before us who were treated successfully on desiccated thyroid. The following represents the hard-earned knowledge of patients who switched to desiccated thyroid, T4/T3 or T3, and regained our health, well-being and bliss. We now give it to you.

1. Some lab work we need; others we don't.

Lab results are extremely important. And patients welcome the extra information the give, since the results can find answers to mysterious symptoms, or help us find our "optimal" dose.

Yet the most unfortunate and egregious mistakes doctors have been making for decades, which has kept us either undiagnosed or undertreated, are two-fold:

1. *To regard the broad "normal ranges" that go with those lab results as being far more important than obvious symptoms, aka clinical presentation*
2. *Failing to understand that it's "where" we fall in those ridiculous ranges that has meaning (especially the free T3 and free T4) not falling just anywhere in them.*

For years, the two lab tests that doctors have worshipped as if they came from God Almighty are the TSH (Thyroid Stimulating Hormone) and the total or Free T4. At the very worst, doctors moved to simply testing the TSH alone...an egregious mistake that has left us sick.

Or they used the outdated and fairly useless "Thyroid Panel", which tests the total T4, the TSH, occasionally the free T4 or total T3, and other lab results such as the Free Thyroxine Index (FTI) or the T3 Resin Uptake (T3RU) or T7 (Addendum C for definitions). Of course, all the latter are good if you want the lab facility to make plenty of money and less of it in your pocket.

We, as patients, have learned that there are certain lab tests which can help us in our assessment of thyroid disease and in our treatment with thyroid medications, as well as where they fall in the range. They include:

- **TSH**
- **Free T4**
- **Free T3**
- **Both Hashimoto's antibodies (TPOab; TgAb)**

Free T3 and Free T4: The *free* in front of the T4 and T3 represents what is available and unbound in the serum by proteins, i.e. what is usable. Without that, labs are only measuring the total hormone, which says nothing about what is usable.

For *diagnosis,* patients have discovered that a free T3 either mid-point or below is often a good confirmation of what symptoms are already telling you. Healthy individuals without a thyroid problem are usually always slightly above midrange! Or, the free T4 can also reveal our hypo- when it's low in its respective range.

When we are optimal on our NDT or T4/T3, the vast majority of us have found our Free T3 at the top part of the range with a mid-range Free T4. Both.

TSH: We have also learned to *only use the TSH to ascertain hypopituitary* (which when not on meds, can be revealed by having a very low TSH along with a low free T3—both and in the presence of raging hypothyroid symptoms).

Granted, you might be the rare patient who finally does have an above-range TSH to help diagnose your hypothyroid to a lab-obsessed doctor. But guess what—that means you've been hypothyroid for awhile! (Chapter 4)

Antibodies: A lot of thyroid patients have antibodies against their own thyroid, which is called Hashimoto's disease. It's important to know, as Hashi's can have more issues to treat than those without it. See the book *Hashimoto's: Taming the Beast.* There are two antibodies in particular:

- **Those targeting your *thyroid peroxidase* (an enzyme that is important in the production of your thyroid hormones).**
- **Those targeting your *thyroglobulin* (a protein carrier for your thyroid hormones).**

It is too common for doctors to state that these antibodies tests are useless (i.e. they see no evidence to order them, even though your symptoms point to Hashi's.) Additionally, we have learned **both are important**, since one can be normal and the other above range. Additionally, knowing you have an autoimmune attack means you can swing between hypo- and hyper- like a pendulum. That latter fact, in turn, can make it useless to dose by lab values! (Chapter 9)

2. Additional lab work can be helpful.

Because hypothyroidism can wreak havoc in our bodies, patients have discovered a whole range of additional lab work which is critical. These include but are not limited to:

- **24-hour cortisol saliva test (requires no prescription)**
- **Full iron panel: serum iron, % saturation, TIBC and ferritin.**
- **B-12**
- **Vitamin D aka 25(OH) and 1,25(OH)—active form**
- **RBC Magnesium, RBC potassium, sodium, calcium, (or a Complete Metabolic Panel)**
- **DHEA**
- **Estrogen**
- **Progesterone**
- **Testosterone**
- **SHBG (Sex Hormone Binding Globulin)**
- **Iodine Loading Test (urine and can be ordered by you)**
- **Reverse T3 (RT3)** ** *See Addendum D about lab tests*

It's rare to see any hypothyroid patient without problems in many of the above. For example, from observations collectively, it appears that **more than 50% of thyroid patients have a cortisol problem,** whether mixed highs and lows, a lot of highs, a lot of lows.

Low iron issues come next in frequency.

Problems in **either** cortisol or iron will always cause issues in raising desiccated thyroid or T4/T3,—iron shoots RT3 up as does high cortisol; low cortisol shoots T3 up, called pooling, because it can't get to the cells without cortisol bringing up blood sugar levels (*Chapters 5 and 6 for adrenals, Chapter 12 for RT3, and Chapter 13 for iron*)

And because of what low iron or cortisol problems do
when you are trying to raise NDT or T3 (anxiety, hyper-
like symptoms, rising RT3, higher BP, worsening hypo),
the NDT is blamed by either the patient or the doctor!
It's not the NDT or T3! It's what they reveal!

**Equally frequent in thyroid patients are inadequate
levels of vitamin D, B12, or even iodine.** Years of
hypothyroidism lead to poor absorption of these nutrients and
more. I also had chronically low levels of both potassium and
magnesium, and sub-optimal levels of D and B12.

Female and male hormonal imbalances come next,
adding to many of our problems. Due to hypothyroid, some
women, but not all, can find themselves with imbalances in
their estrogen and progesterone, as well as testosterone levels.
Some have problems getting pregnant. Some bleed too heavily
in menstruation. Some enter menopause too early.

Hypothyroid decreases SHBG—a protein which carries
testosterone and some estrogen through the body. The latter
can cause hormonal swings. The symptoms of any of the above
sex hormone imbalances can also mimic hypothyroid symptoms.

Ask your doctor for other lab test recommendations, like the
Epstein Barr Virus, which can reactivate due to emotional or
physical stress.

3. The right amount of cortisol helps us raise our thyroid meds with problems.

Remarkably, we have discovered that a large percentage of
thyroid patients have either dysfunctional adrenal function,
or sluggishness, also called adrenal fatigue—all due to being
undiagnosed thanks to the lousy TSH, or put on T4-only meds,
or being underdosed. Even a constant attack on the thyroid
with Hashimoto's can mess up our cortisol.

Cortisol issues, as revealed by saliva cortisol testing, range
from **1) a mix of high and low cortisol 2) mostly high cortisol. or
3) mostly low**. In healthy situations, cortisol is released by your
adrenals to help you cope with stress, besides playing a role
in facilitating the thyroid receptors on your cells in receiving

without cortisol regulating rhythm, T3 [cannot] get into cells

the thyroid hormones from your blood. But our levels can get
messed up due to the stress of our thyroid situation. *See p. 47*

The consequences of erratic cortisol production are profound
for thyroid patients. Not only do you lack the ability to
appropriately cope with stress, you lose the success of raising
your desiccated thyroid or T4/T3 to optimal levels. Thyroid
hormones, especially T3, will build high in your blood rather
than make it to your cells, which we term "pooling". You will
also have hyper-like symptoms and misery as you try to raise
desiccated thyroid or T3. (Chapter 5)

Why do so many thyroid patients have an adrenal problem?
We can surmise that years of being undiagnosed due to doctors'
over-reliance on faulty labs and cheesy normal ranges, years
of the stress of the thyroid attack for Hashimoto's patients,
followed by poor treatment with levothyroxine or other T4-
only medications, have played a role in the overworking
of our stress-busting adrenals to make up for the slack. To
the degree that your hypothyroid condition continues, to the
same degree and ten-fold your adrenals try to make up the
slack, then they become exhausted.

Additionally, we can surmise that chemicals we are
exposed to daily in plastics, food and water—including but
not limited to fluoride, bromide and more, may have played
a taxing role in the chronic stress on our adrenals. Add to
that the emotional stress of our modern lives and you have
a recipe for disaster for your adrenals.

Thus, at the beginning of our thyroid diagnosis or
treatment, we have found it wise to learn the status
of our adrenal cortisol production. Chapter Five gives
you Discovery Steps to help you discern if you have
adrenal problem. Discovery Step One asks you pertinent
questions. Discovery Two explains certain tests you can
do in the privacy of your own home. If either or both are
suspicious, it can be time to consider a 24-hour cortisol
saliva test, which unlike a one-time blood test commonly
prescribed by doctors, will test your cellular cortisol levels
are four key times during a 24-hour period (or six with
some facilities, but honestly not as necessary). It doesn't

require a prescription, and it's less stressful since you do it in your own home. (Addendum D for places to get your cortisol tested with saliva.)

The ACTH STIM test is commonly prescribed by doctors if you suggest you may have an adrenal problem. ACTH is the hormone secreted by your pituitary with the purpose of motivating your adrenals. But most patients have found themselves with normal ACTH results, even when the saliva test revealed otherwise. Your ACTH may be normal, but your adrenals too sluggish to perform. (Chapter 5.)

The 24-hour urine test can also prove to be inadequate, since it takes the average of a total day's production of cortisol, leaving you clueless as to what specifically is going on with your adrenals at specific times of the day.

If we find ourselves with cortisol issues, treatment ranges from the use of adaptogens (for healthy function but stressed), to over-the-counter adrenal cortex or prescription HC (for too many lows). If cortisol levels are overall too high, you need to work to lower it. Chapter 6 covers this topic.

4. There are successful ways to transition from T4 to desiccated thyroid.

When making a switch to desiccated thyroid, we and certain wise doctors have found two successful strategies: first, to take our last dose of T4 (aka Synthroid, Levoxyl, Levothyroxine, etc.) one day, and start on a safe dose of natural desiccated thyroid the next, as explained below.

Or second, a patient can lower her T4 dose in half, and start on desiccated thyroid. But it will be important to continue lowering the T4 with each raise of desiccated thyroid to prevent an excess of T4. Most desiccated thyroid is 80% T4 anyway! The latter is why it become problematic to keep T4 along with NDT!

With transitioning to the two synthetics (T4/T3), we just lower the T4 a bit, then in add in T3, starting low and building, and checking the frees.

5. We learned safe ways to start on and to raise our desiccated thyroid.

Generally, we and informed doctors have found that a safe dose to start on is around one grain, which equates to 60 or 65 mg depending on the brand used. Some may need to start lower due to heart issues, excessively low cortisol, or other conditions. Some can start a little higher, but one grain has been our experience as a safe introductory amount for most.

--->*For me, starting on a safer lower dose was very important due to having a benign heart condition called Mitral Valve Prolapse (MVP). My mitral valve always proves itself to be very sensitive to certain substances or changes. So, it was important for me to start as low as one grain to allow my sensitive valve to adjust to the direct T3, which my body was starved for, and to raise in small amounts every week or two. I had heart palpitations when I started desiccated thyroid and with every raise, but they always subsided within a few days. After I was optimal, I rarely have any palps for any reason! This adjustment to the direct T3 can be important for your entire body.*

Once patients start on one grain, we and some of our best doctors have learned to hold that amount 'up to' two weeks--- though some might need to go up a little sooner if symptoms return too quickly. We are raising by approximately ½ grain in the same way---in 'up to' two weeks. For many of us, if we stay on that introductory dose too long, our hypothyroid symptoms start to return with a vengeance due to the negative feedback loop between the hypothalamus, pituitary and thyroid gland. The individuality is when it will happen.

Then for most of us, we do our next lab work (free T3 and free T4) somewhere in the 2-3-grain, making sure we've been on that dose a few weeks before testing to show its T4-to-T3 conversion results.

It appears that a large body of patients on the continuum of doses end up needing 3-5 grains, which may be closely equivalent to the amount that a healthy thyroid might be making[10]. Some might need less to be optimal, such as somewhere in the

---

[10] https://www.thyroidmanager.org/chapter/chapter-2-thyroid-hormone-synthesis-and-secretion/

2 grains area. Occasionally, some doctors find their patients needing even more than 5 grains when an optimal dose is found, as mentioned below. And of course, it's individual, since we occasionally see some patients optimal at slightly less than 3 grains. No matter what the dose, **optimal** is our goal.

6. To find our optimal dose of desiccated thyroid, we seek all three criteria below.

- A mid-afternoon consistent temperature close to 98.6F/ 37C, using a mercury or liquid thermometer, along with normal blood pressure and heart rate. For females still having periods, only done before ovulation.
- The complete or near-complete elimination of our hypo-thyroid symptoms and which lasts—doesn't go away.
- The most important: A free T3 towards the top part of the range, and a free T4 around midrange—both, no matter how low the TSH will plunge. *Note: having a free T3 at the top of the range, if not over, in the presence of continuing hypo- symptoms, is a clue you may have adrenal issues. It's called "pooling", meaning the T3 isn't getting to the cells due to a cortisol problem.*

Dosing by the elimination symptoms was done for decades before most labs came into existence. But watching the frees is also critically important, as we have seen that we will feel good before we are optimal, and it backfires if we aren't optimal! We also make sure we do not take desiccated thyroid or T3 before our labs, which only results in a false high reading.

7. We have learned that symptoms diminish with each raise of our NDT or T3.

It's very individual, but some of the first improvements we see as we raise our natural desiccated thyroid include the softening of our hair and skin, lessening of our brain fog, and better energy. As we continue, our depression lifts, and aches and pains cease, and our cholesterol falls. Gone is the fatigue that was once classified as the mysterious Chronic Fatigue Syndrome (in lieu of having Lyme Disease, acute EBV, etc.). It gives back the stamina that we never had. We see an improvement in our bone density and strengthening of our heart muscle.

Raising our desiccated thyroid or T3 to *optimal* improves or removes our chronic headaches (in the presence of strong adrenals) and improves our female hormonal issues. It helps us get pregnant when that goal is desired. It stops our hair loss and slowly allows new growth to come back in. It gives us back our sanity. Optimal NDT can even lower Hashi's antibodies in some.

Note that all the above occurs in the presence of healthy adrenal function, good iron levels, and correct treatment for either. Without good levels, we have problems with raising.

8. Problems that arise when on desiccated thyroid (or T3) are correctable.

For those of us who have had problems with desiccated thyroid, it was due to four correctable issues, in most cases:

- **Being held on low introductory doses far too long, allowing our hypo to return with a vengeance.** We and wise doctors have learned NOT to stay on an introductory dose much longer than two weeks or less before raising. This can be challenging if you have a doctor who expects you to wait 6-8 weeks and more until your next appointment.
- **Being held hostage to the unreliable TSH lab value.** Since the TSH and its dubious "normal" range can and has failed us, we dose by the free T4 and free T3, *NOT* the TSH. As we seek our optimal dose of our thyroid meds with T3 in them, it is perfectly normal for the TSH to go below range. And to the contrary as doctors exclaim, it does not cause bone loss or heart problems!! They confuse it with Graves' disease which tanks the TSH.
- **Failing to recognize the problem of cortisol issues or inadequate iron when trying to raise our thyroid meds.** The right amount of cortisol is needed to raise blood sugar

levels in our cells, which in turn interacts with T3. And without healthy cortisol release, problems develop when raising thyroid meds that resemble hyper symptoms, such as *anxiety, shakiness, nausea, sleep issues, feeling hot, etc.* Cortisol problems (too low most of the time) result in a high free T3 with continuing hypo- symptoms, called pooling, meaning not getting to the cells well. High cortisol can push RT3 up (reverse T3), which will make us more hypo. Depending on results of saliva cortisol, we then choose either adaptogens several times a day (for minor issues or a seesaw high and low mix), or over-the-counter Adrenal Cortex (for moderate low cortisol), or prescription cortisol, aka Cortef (Hydrocortisone or HC) for more serious low cortisol. Once we have found our optimal dose of cortisol by using our Daily Average Temps comparisons, we can then continue with raising our desiccated thyroid, or T3, while on adrenal support. (Chapter 6)

- **Having inadequate iron levels.** Because of digestive issues or low stomach acid from being hypothyroid, having inadequate levels of iron is common among thyroid patients, as discovered by the serum iron test. Low serum iron can cause problems as we try to raise desiccated thyroid, besides give us symptoms resembling hypothyroid if levels are low enough. We then supplement with up to 150-200 mg "elemental iron" daily in tablets (less in liquid iron, since it's highly absorbable), taken with food and Vitamin C—the latter to counter free radicals. Improving low levels can take 8 weeks minimum. *If ferritin (storage iron) looks high, it can point to inflammation, which causes iron to be thrust into storage. (Chapter 13.)*

9. Desiccated thyroid seems to work best when we multi-dose. Sublingual, under the tongue, has worked for some brands.

Since a healthy thyroid produces hormones as needed throughout the day, we emulate that by multi-dosing our desiccated thyroid rather than taking it in one big dose in the morning, which not only puts too much T3 in the body at once, but might leave you sleepy in the late afternoon. We all experiment to find what works best for us, and generally, that means taking *the highest amount in the morning, followed by a lower amount in the early afternoon.* Or, we can take three doses–morning, early afternoon, late afternoon, etc., but not usually necessary. Some even take a final very small dose at bedtime. Since the direct T3 in desiccated thyroid peaks about two hours after you take it, multi-dosing prevents a huge spike, which can be hard on our adrenals.

Some brands of desiccated thyroid can be done sublingually (under the tongue) due to the higher dextrose amount or lack of hard coating. Acella's NP Thyroid is one: Erfa in Canada may be another. It's direct and immediate, and enzymes in saliva are breaking it down for better absorption, as well. In other words, you get more of what you give yourself by doing the desiccated thyroid sublingually rather than swallowing. T3 can often be done that way, too, for those on the two synthetics.

This does not mean you can't swallow your desiccated thyroid and get benefits. Some patients prefer swallowing, and still get benefits! But if you do swallow, avoid swallowing calcium, iron, high fiber and estrogen with it to prevent the, binding of 'some' of the thyroid hormones as they mix in your stomach. On a positive side, swallowing desiccated thyroid (or T3) with food slows the release of the thyroid hormones to your body, distributing it better throughout the day.

Note: if any brand seems especially hard or with a tough coating, chewing the tablet up before swallowing helps release the thyroid hormones.

10. We learned <u>not</u> to take our desiccated thyroid before morning lab work.

The direct T3 found in desiccated thyroid peaks approximately two hours minimum after we swallow or take it sublingually, and with a slow decline, causing our free T3 lab result to look high and give a false impression of hyper to doctors who are obsessed with lab work. Thus, we have found it wise to avoid taking any desiccated thyroid before we do our scheduled labs. In other words, we take our final dose the day before, and refrain from doing our morning dose until we can get our labs done. This refrain from taking desiccated thyroid can also be true for saliva tests, where you should only swallow it after the morning spit and the noon spit, for example.

11. Wintertime or intense activity can heighten our need for a bit more desiccated thyroid.

If we are frequently exposed to cold air during the winter, we have learned that it can be wise to add a slight amount of desiccated thyroid, such as ¼ grain, to our daily optimal dose. This slight dose raise can also be true if we participate in a strenuous activity in any season of the year, since the activity can increase the need for the direct T3. If we are on needed adrenal support, a strenuous activity, stress or illness can dictate the need for a bit extra cortisol, as well.

12. Good doctors can be hard to come by, but we look for certain attributes.

Generally, we as thyroid patients have experienced that a large body of our doctors have been unwilling to help us achieve optimal thyroid treatment—they are paranoid about the low TSH. We have experienced many to be excessively rigid about prescribing T4-only medications, ignorant or close-minded about desiccated thyroid or adrenal problems, disrespectful about our own knowledge about our bodies, and too obsessed with lab work like the TSH rather than listening to the clinical presentation of our symptoms.

Additionally, we have repeatedly found endocrinologists to be the least open-minded, besides rigid about the TSH and thyroxine medications. There are exceptions, but few.

We have learned to find a doctor who is open about the use of desiccated thyroid or T4/T3, helps us go by the free T4 and free T3 and being "optimal", and who will listen about adrenal and iron issues causing problems. We also value doctors who work with us as a team, respecting our own wisdom since we live in our bodies, and our own knowledge via research and reading important books like this one.

13. Iodine may be a beneficial supplement

Many patients use Lugols, a liquid form, either topically or with drops into juice or water, or Iodoral, a pill form. Moving up to 50 mg has been a recommended dose, but others stay much lower in the iodine amount, especially with Hashimoto's disease. The use of iodine helps eliminate toxins from your body, especially bromide. This toxin release can produce symptoms such as fatigue, pimples, or a headache, or can make Hashimoto's worse. The recommended solution is taking supporting nutrients such as minerals like selenium and magnesium, as well as Vitamin C, sea salt and more, plus going *low and slow.*

Hashimoto's patients, as well as adrenal patients, have reported both negative and positive experiences with iodine, ranging from an increase of antibodies, to further stress on one's adrenals. This is why we've learned to go low and slow if one has Hashimoto's.

On the positive side (!), other patients who used iodine have had very positive experiences, from a lowering of antibodies, to better adrenal function. For women, iodine use has removed fibrocystic breast disease. They key may be the use of the supporting nutrients mentioned above, and going low and slow.

Because patients are still learning about iodine use, I highly recommend that patients do their own research to make an informed decision.

14. We have learned to be our own best advocates.

In previous generations, and including our own, it's been common to look at the doctor as an extension of God Almighty: my doctor knows what's best; my doctor will tell me what to do; my doctor can figure out what is going on; my doctor knows more than I know; my doctor will do the right thing to make me well. **Most all of us have spent years entering our doctor's offices and giving our power away!**

But thyroid patients have learned to walk into that office knowledgeable (which this book will help you do), and to expect the relationship to be a team—the doctor's expertise *and your own intelligence, wisdom and intuitive knowledge since you live in your body.* This has become especially crucial for thyroid patients in light of local doctors who may know little about desiccated thyroid, sluggish adrenals, or not understanding how to read lab work!

THINGS WE HAVE LEARNED TIDBITS

* It is common to "feel good" before we are optimal, and patients make the mistake of stopping there. Thus, it eventually backfires. Being optimal is important.

* Much of this information can apply to using T4 with T3.

* We take our meds as usual one day (except in the evenings), then do labs the next morning without taking our meds before labs.

Chapter 4

TSH: THYROID STIMULATING HOOEY AKA, WHY YOU MAY STILL BE HYPOTHYROID WITH A NORMAL TSH

t's probably one of the most commonly prescribed lab tests worldwide—the Thyroid Stimulating Hormone, aka TSH test or thyrotropin. In fact, talk to your endocrinologist or most any medical-school-trained doctor, and you will be told the TSH lab test is *a reliable gauge of your thyroid function, i.e. whether you are hypo-, hyper-, or normal.* The same doctors would also state that the TSH lab is an accurate guide to determine the right dose of thyroid medications. Even the most prestigious medical websites and journals will state the same. And it's a pronouncement which has been going on for years. **But, experiences of patients have found both of the above TSH pronouncements (reliable physiologic marker and accurate dosing guide) to be totally and unequivocally false!**

In fact, it's too common to see the majority of thyroid patients, who have obvious and classic hypothyroid symptoms, report that a doctor pronounced them *"normal"* for years because of a TSH lab result which fell between the two man-made parameters of the so-called "normal" range, which might be the old 0.5 - 5.0, the 0.3 - 3.0, or even much higher as in the UK!! The end result? The doctor's overt reliance on the TSH test and its dubious range browbeats us into believing that we must be crazy, hypochondriac, or at the very least, just plain ol' mistaken.

Cough.

Finally, after years go by... voila! That ink spot on the piece of paper confirms what our symptoms told us for years anyway. But patients' question: *Where is the victory in the diagnosis when they had to suffer for so long? Where is the victory when we might now have low cortisol, low iron?*

Joan noticed she needed afternoon naps after her normal pre-lunch bike rides, whereas before, her energy levels were high enough to ride again in the afternoon. Concerned, she made an appointment with her family doctor, who first sent her to do the TSH lab work.

> *"When I sat down in his office and went over my fatigue, he outright dismissed it, telling me I simply may be pregnant. Pregnant!! I was single and had not had a relationship with anyone for months! When I asked about my lab results, he just looked at me and said everything was normal. Wait a minute. It was normal to need naps that I hadn't needed before?? I was confused, but he was the "expert". And it took me four more years of a "normal" TSH lab test and losing my ability to ride my bike without consequences before he diagnosed me as "borderline" hypothyroid."*

Joan's story of being undiagnosed for years due to the TSH lab is so common that it reeks of scandal. In fact, I have observed many a patient who clearly had symptoms of hypothyroid for years before their TSH lab result even came close to clueing in their symptom-blind doctors.

What is the TSH?

In your body, there's a feedback loop called thyroid-pituitary-hypothalamic axis, where the hypothalamus messages the pituitary, then the pituitary releases the messenger hormones TSH to knock on the door the thyroid to produce.

If activity or illness increases your body's demands for assistance from your thyroid, the messenger will knock on the door a bit harder. If you have an excess of thyroid hormones when you don't need them, the messenger will knock much lighter.

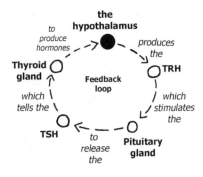

But when your thyroid gland becomes diseased or disabled and fails to do its job adequately, the TSH knocks and knocks on the door, and theoretically, the TSH lab will show a consistently high number. Or, if the thyroid gland gets on its exercise bicycle and overproduces thyroid hormones (called hyperthyroid), the TSH lab will theoretically go low to indicate that the TSH in your body isn't knocking.

Yet patients have found the TSH lab to be a poor reflection of the reality of their thyroid condition, most especially for hypothyroid! It lags behind!! Additionally, when a thyroid patient has the autoimmune thyroid disease called Hashimoto's, the TSH, just like the free T3 and free T4, can move all over the place in response to the die-off of the attacked thyroid. And you're out of luck if you have your blood drawn during one of the low-normal swings of your TSH.

The creation of the TSH lab

The TSH lab test was developed around 1973, using a base of select volunteers with no presumed history of thyroid disease to establish the "normal" range. Over the years, additional population studies have been done to support the range. The "normal" reference range is intended to represent the range of values for those in a healthy population without any presumed thyroid problem. The lowest and highest readings used to create the range are usually thrown out.

Dr. David Derry, a renowned physician in Canada, had been practicing medicine just two years when the TSH lab was introduced. In an interview[11], he stated he was able to watch whether the TSH was in line with the onset of hypothyroidism. And he came to the conclusion that it was either quite slow to reveal it, or didn't at all. Dr. Derry discovered exactly what we, as patients, have experienced for five decades–*the TSH lab result is thoroughly unrelated to how we feel!*

Does the TSH lab have a role when we are on thyroid medications? From the experience of patients, the answer is a resounding NO!

Sure, the vast majority of us have been dosed according to the TSH lab result. Our doctors have told us for years that because our result was in a particular place in the reference range, we were now on a correct amount of thyroid medications and adequately treated.

But patients who have switched to desiccated thyroid have discovered that when they are allowed to dose to achieve an *optimal free T3 and free T4*, they end up with a TSH value very below range...and not one hint of hyperthyroid. It is not uncommon to see a TSH of 0.009 or 0.004 when optimal, for example, yet not one iota of hyper, and no underlying problems with our hearts or of osteoporosis–the latter which uninformed doctors will declare.

Here is an example of lab work for an individual who had what appeared to be a very normal and optimal TSH. Yet, the patient made it clear that she continued to have hypothyroid symptoms of poor stamina, afternoon fatigue, hair loss and constipation. Additionally, when you view the free T3 and free T4, you will see the dead giveaway of the continuing hypothyroid condition, as both numbers are at the low end of each range:

- Free T3 2.65 *(2.00 - 4.20 pg/mL)*
- Free T4 0.89 *(0.71 - 1.85 ug/dL)*
- TSH 1.58 *(0.35 - 4.00 ug/mL)*

---

[11] www.thyroid-info.com/articles/david-derry.htm

The answer as to why the TSH lab can be so counter to how we feel lies in our tissues. Each of our organs will independently manage the amount of thyroid hormones which are received into its tissues via the conversion of T4 to T3 by enzymes, especially the liver and the brain. In other words, though one organ achieves optimal T3 from conversion, another organ will not. And the organ that is not getting enough T3 has no way to tell the thyroid that it needs more.

A report in 2005 from the Athens University School of Medicine[12], stated it this way:

> *Conversion of T4 to T3 is greater in the pituitary than in the liver, therefore it is possible that euthyroidism [without hypothyroid symptoms] in pituitary cells may co-exist with hypothyroidism in liver cells.*

When Dr. John C. Lowe wrote his classic *Addenda to Four 2003 Studies of Thyroid Hormone Replacement Therapies,* he stated tissue responsiveness to thyroid hormone dosages can vary widely among patients.

Where the TSH lab can be useful: hypopituitary

In spite of the worldwide patient experience with the TSH as a lousy test for hypothyroid diagnosing and dosing, there is one area where it can be quite useful: to discern pituitary function. Occasionally, a patient will have a very low TSH lab result with raging or classic hypothyroid symptoms, and that can point to a problem in the pituitary gland, which normally secretes the TSH hormone. This failure is called Hypopituitary.

Hypopituitarism is where your pituitary gland fails to produce enough, or any of, important messenger hormones. This causes a domino-like downward effect in your health.

Pituitary hormones include the **TSH** (stimulates your thyroid to produce); the **ACTH** (stimulates your adrenals to produce cortisol); the **FSH and LH** (influences the testes and

---

[12] www.springerlink.com/content/y28n557300582h33/

ovaries in the production of testosterone and estrogen); the **GH** growth hormone (promotes normal growth of your bones and tissue); the **ADH** antidiuretic hormone (helps control the water loss by your kidneys); and the **prolactin** hormone, which stimulates milk production and female breast growth.

The condition has many causes, including an injury to the head, excessive blood loss (especially from childbirth or an injury), a disease in the gland itself, meningitis, or a problem with the hypothalamus, which is the organ that sends its hormone messenger to the pituitary. I frequently note that many with a previous head injury develop hypopituitary later, even if not all.

Treatment involves replacing hormones from those glands the pituitary fails to stimulate, or treating the underlying cause of the sluggish pituitary state.

Smoking and your TSH

From a study done in Norway in 2006[13], there is evidence that the stimulating effect of smoking can lower your TSH lab result. So, if your doctor is still attached to the TSH lab, and you know you have hypothyroid symptoms, it may be wise to avoid smoking the day of your lab work if not the day before, as well as avoid second-hand smoke.

The bottom line about the TSH lab according to the experience of patients

For the thyroid patient report card, it sucks.

The TSH lab can be affected by too many variables! These can include an autoimmune attack on your thyroid (causing you to swing between hypo- and hyper), your daily hormonal ebb and flow, the weather, numerous medical conditions, getting older, infections, or can just plan lag behind what is really going on with you for years. And, there are simply a large percentage of hypothyroid patients who have continuing hypothyroid symptoms with a TSH lab result in the "normal" range and for years!

---

[13] https://www.ncbi.nlm.nih.gov/pubmed/16915535

Our recommendations to our doctors?

Pay attention to our symptoms, then use the free T3 and free T4, seeking optimal placement in the ranges, plus the two antibodies tests, as adjuncts to the clinical presentation of our hypothyroid! See Addendum C for explanations of thyroid labs.

The grandest use for the TSH lab test pertains to what it is: a pituitary hormone...no more, no less. And for that, the TSH lab is a good guide to reveal if you have a *malfunctioning pituitary gland*, especially if you have a very low TSH with a low free T3, accompanied by raging hypothyroid symptoms.

For the prompt diagnosis of a thyroid condition, as well as finding the optimal amount of thyroid medications, patients give a resounding "Useless!" to the TSH lab.

STOP DIAGNOSING OR DOSING US BY THE USELESS TSH TEST!!

TSH TIDBITS

* A TSH can be at its lowest around noon, and highest during the night.

* TSH is a pituitary hormone, not a thyroid hormone, and can never reveal whether all parts of your body are getting enough thyroid hormones.

* When we are optimal with our frees (Free T3 at the top part of the range; Free T4 midrange), it's very normal for the TSH to be below range. That is NOT the same as Graves' disease, which also tanks the TSH. We do NOT have bone loss, or heart disease, from our low TSH.

Chapter 5

DON'T IGNORE YOUR ADRENAL GLANDS: THE MONKEY WRENCH IN THE WORKS

J ust when you think you've gotten ahead of the game with your new knowledge about better thyroid treatment, a new stumbling block can rear its ugly head for many thyroid patients: *adrenal problems, going from high cortisol, then mixed high and low, then low cortisol.*

In fact, it's been my observation that at least 50% of hypothyroid patients may have an adrena̶ And without discovering and treating that potenti̶ you will be unable to benefit from your better thy̶ ent. Why? Because cortisol issues can block conversion of T4 to T3, besides closing the door to cell reception of thyroid hormones due to low cellular level of glucose from low cortisol.

Healthy adrenals and how they can turn on you

Your adrenals are walnut-sized glands which sit atop your kidneys. Like your thyroid, they are cued into action by the communications from the hypothalamus to the pituitary gland to the adrenals (HPA axis releasing the ACTH). When your adrenal glands and HPA axis are healthy and strong, the adrenals have a powerful biological role of helping you cope with stress, whether physical, emotional, or mental. It's a process you may not even realize is going on, so you take it for granted. But they are like an invisible knight-protector who's ready to absorb or squelch any stressful blows from life's dragons.

In response to stress, your adrenals produce two key hormones to help you cope: **adrenaline**, which plays a role in your short-term reaction to stress, and **cortisol**, which has a longer action and a variety of stress-busting roles. Cortisol is a "glucocorticoid" hormone. The "gluco" refers to the fact that it stimulates your levels of blood sugar (glucose) and the "corticoid" means it's released by the adrenal cortex part of the gland.

Your adrenals also produce **aldosterone**, which helps maintain your internal fluid balance and blood pressure, and the sex hormones testosterone as well as DHEA. And key for thyroid patients, it's the adrenal hormone cortisol which helps all run smoothly.

Unfortunately, adrenals can fall off their horse and fail to help you. Below are three common scenarios which can result in problem:

1. Being on a T4-only treatment like Synthroid, Eltroxin, levothyroxine or other brands *(which leaves you hypothyroid, causes your adrenals to take up the slack, and eventually decreases the health of your adrenals which need T3.)*

2. Spending years being undiagnosed as hypothyroid due to your doctor's rigid dependence on the unreliable TSH lab with its dubious normal range

3. Enduring long periods of chronic stress---biological, emotional, or physical *(which causes your adrenals to overwork, reserves to be depleted, and can be an additional burden if you also have the former two scenarios).*

4. Eating improperly such as a high carbohydrate diet with low fat; consuming excess toxins in fluoridated and chlorinated water.

The tell-tale signs of adrenal stress

One of the first clues that your adrenals are overly challenged, dysfunctional and/or becoming fatigued can be a cluster of symptoms you've noticed before you even got on desiccated thyroid medication, or when you are trying to raise your desiccated thyroid:

- Anxiety
- Nervousness
- Not coping well with stress
- Impatience, irritability with others
- Feeling light-headed
- Shaky or trembling
- Dizziness
- Racing or pounding heart
- Trouble sleeping at night
- Nausea or feeling hot in the face of stress
- Hypoglycemia (low blood sugar)
- Sweating
- Salt craving; Sweet craving

Some patients with adrenal stress may start on desiccated thyroid or T3 without an issue. But they can also notice fairly quickly, or after moving up on the dose, that something is not quite right. Namely, you might notice symptoms that seem like an overreaction to your medication similar to feeling hyper. I'll never forget Julie, an author of children's books, who had a bad reaction when she reached 90 mg. She recounted:

I sure was excited when I found out about natural desiccated thyroid. My eleven-year use of Levo had done practically nothing for me. Yeah it was a little better than before I started, but I still had problems. And my continued symptoms were affecting my ability to write, which of course my doctor said was because of depression. I also became a recluse, which really bothered my husband and son. And my friends weren't too pleased with that, either. When I first started on NDT, I had such hope! I did feel better. But on the day I was ready to raise to 1 ½ grains (90 mg), I became breathless and my heart felt like it was going to beat out of my chest. I also had this strange tight feeling in my chest. And my anxiety was huge! I felt like I was going to crawl out of my skin.

Julie's story is common to many patients who are started on desiccated thyroid with their doctors being clueless about their adrenal situation. Strange reactions occur, causing thyroid patients to think they are allergic to desiccated thyroid, or sensitive, *or "NDT isn't right for me!"* Some experience it on lower doses; some on higher doses.

Another common scenario with adrenal problems while on desiccated thyroid is a free T3 lab result high or over-range with continuing hypo- symptoms (thyroid hormone failure to get to the cells called **pooling**), or a high free T4 and low free T3 (with excess Reverse T3). In either situation, your clueless doctor thinks you simply need to lower your meds, or add more T4. i.e. your well- meaning doctor fails to put the adrenal puzzle pieces together.

Patients putting it all together

Finally, as patients talked in groups, researched on the internet, and talked to or read the words of the few knowledgeable doctors out there, light bulbs began to light in our brains about all the above. No more would we need to exclaim *"Desiccated thyroid doesn't work for me!"* or listen to doctors adamantly stating the same. We recognized that the strange problems we were experiencing before we started on desiccated thyroid, or after we started, were due to the highs and lows of stressed cortisol production and its bad effect on thyroid hormone assimilation.

Thierry Hertoghe, in *The International Hormone Society's Consensus Group statement*[14] states:

> *The intolerance may come from over activity of the orthosympathic nervous system that often accompanies states of low cortisol, and an excessive and rapid conversion of thyroxin to triiodothyronine that puts these patients*

[14] http://intlhormonesociety.org/index.php?option=com_content&task=view&id=31 &Itemid=53

*easily into a state of excess T3 and thus hyperthyroidism,
and further increases the orthosympathic activity.*

But patient experience actually suggests that the symptoms
are caused by an excess of adrenaline rather than just the high
T3, followed by conversion to an excess of Reverse T3 and its
problems with cell reception.

We could sum it up in two sentences:

1. *Adequate or proper levels of cortisol are crucial
   when you start on, or are raising, desiccated
   thyroid or any product with T3.*
2. *Without those healthy levels of cortisol, problems
   will ensue!*

Why some doctors haven't pointed out our adrenal problems

When you look at the medical school training of the
majority of doctors, you'll find out that the books accentuate
Addison's disease or Cushing's syndrome—the extreme low and
the overtly high of dysfunctional cortisol output. Addison's,
named after the English physician who first identified the
disease in an 1855 publication, is a progressive destruction of
the glands, and is most commonly caused by an autoimmune
attack. Technically, you will see the term *adrenal insufficiency*
used to describe the effects of Addison's disease.

On the other side of the coin, our adrenal problem is more
aptly described as *adrenal (or HPA) dysfunction*, since it's more
of a dysfunction or sluggishness than a disease process. It can
also result in both high and low cortisol as well as cortisol
resistance, all at the same time. Some can fall into Addison's-
type levels (not having Addison's, but having quite low levels
like Addison's) while others stay in an adrenal limbo. And our
different, yet still highly problematic variety of an adrenal
problem, has been missed by our doctors. In fact, it's most likely
far more common and widespread to be missed.

Additionally, with our doctors' *blind and zombie faith in
T4-only medications and the TSH lab test,* and their failure to
give credence to our years and years of coping with continued

hypothyroid symptoms, it has probably not even dawned on them what has been occurring. *It's the blind leading the blind.* If we do get a miracle and our doctors prescribe desiccated thyroid, they even seem to miss what is written in the prescribing information for Armour by Forest Laboratories, Inc, for example:

> *Thyroid hormone preparations are generally contraindicated in patients with diagnosed, but as yet uncorrected, adrenal cortical insufficiency...*

James L. Wilson, N.D., in his book *Adrenal Fatigue, The 21st Century Stress Syndrome,* further adds that in addition to their lack of training, *medical doctors of today are constricted by medical licensing boards, the health insurance and pharmaceutical industries, and their patient's expectations of quick recovery*[15].

When a doctor does recognize the adrenal factor, he or she might describe the adrenal dysfunction experienced by hypothyroid patients as a "mild deficiency" since it's not as grave as Addison's disease with its autoimmune devastation of the adrenal cortex. The adrenal problem experienced by hypothyroid patients, on the other hand, is a dysfunctional mix of producing too much cortisol some of the day, and too little at other times. *And this causes innumerable problems that no patient would call "mild."*

Other factors contributing to our adrenal fatigue

As thyroid patients, we have also surmised that the excessive amounts of added fluoride and chlorine in the public water supply may have contributed to the cascade that leads to stressed adrenals. Fluoride, as a man-made chemical added to our water, toothpastes and certain foods and beverages is a known thyroid depressor, even used decades ago to treat *hyper*thyroidism. So, our lowered T3 levels end up stressing our adrenals.

---

[15] Page 52

Additionally, who knows what effect the mercury in our vaccines and fillings, bromine in pesticides and foods, plastics in drinking bottles, and pollutants like PCB's and pharmaceutical residues which have leeched into our water supply have played in the stress on our adrenals. Repeated and extended periods of an excessively demanding life can further the stress on our adrenals as they attempt to help us cope. These stressors increase our nutritional needs, and those needs may not be met by our propensity to eat excessive carbohydrates.

Adrenal fatigue as an HPA dysfunction

Though "adrenal fatigue" is a common term to describe a low cortisol condition, it may go deeper than it sounds. That depth was proposed to us by Dr. Kent Holtorf in his paper titled *Diagnosis and Treatment of Hypothalamic-Pituitary-Adrenal (HPA) Axis Dysfunction in Patients with Chronic Fatigue Syndrome (CFS) and Fibromyalgia (FM)* (Journal of Chronic Fatigue Syndrome Vol 14:3 2008). Holtorf suspects a sluggish HPA axis (communication from the hypothalamus, to the pituitary, to the adrenal glands) is the problem, even if the exact dysfunction is not known. Look at the HPA axis like a perfect human Rube Goldberg machine of chain reactions, which if not working properly, affects the healthy actions of other organs, including your thyroid, adrenals and sex hormones.

Bottom line, a significant body of thyroid patients find themselves with low-functioning adrenal glands, with the resultant low cortisol, complicating their hypothyroid condition.

Two kinds of our adrenal fatigue:
Primary and Secondary

Ongoing hypothyroidism because of T4-only treatment and the use of the lousy TSH lab test, as well as being underdosed, all contribute to what is called *Primary Adrenal Fatigue,* or the inadequate secretion of cortisol by your adrenals, in spite of normal or high levels of ACTH (Adrenocorticotropic hormone) knocking on its door from the pituitary. (*Primary Adrenal "Insufficiency"* is the term applied to Addison's disease, usually from an autoimmune attack or even tuberculosis.)

Secondary Adrenal Fatigue is the result of a failure of the pituitary gland to send the ACTH messenger, also called *Hypopituitarism*. It has a variety of causes, from a head injury, excessive blood loss, a tumor on the pituitary gland, and a viral implication...to having antibodies against the pituitary. It's usually detected when you have low cortisol or thyroid levels, and a low serum ACTH. In many cases, it can have no cure and require supplementation of the missing hormones for life.

The full list of adrenal dysfunction symptoms

On a previous page of this chapter, I listed tell-tale signs of having an adrenal problem. There are even more to consider below. The following is a more complete list of actual low cortisol symptoms reported by patients who had confirmed adrenal issues, whether primary or secondary, and many with mixed levels of high and low. And some of these symptoms, especially the shaky sensation, can be the result of the over-production of adrenaline by your adrenals in the presence of low cortisol:

- continuing hypo- symptoms with a high free T3
- shaky hands; internal feeling of shakiness
- diarrhea
- heart palpitations
- feeling of doom or panic
- irrational fear
- general or localized weakness
- inability to handle stress
- social interactions problems
- inability to focus
- rage or sudden angry outbursts
- emotionally hypersensitive
- overreactive
- highly defensive
- paranoid
- no patience
- easily irritated
- mild to severe hypoglycemia
- slow recovery from stress
- slow recovery from dental work

- flu-like symptoms
- headaches
- all-over body ache
- chronic inflammation
- super-sensitive skin
- clumsy
- sudden extreme hunger
- hypersensitive to supplements
- low stomach acid
- low back pain
- feeling dull
- cloud-filled head
- jumpiness
- muscle weakness
- dizziness
- light-headedness
- motion sickness
- coffee sleepiness
- dependence on morning coffee
- incline vom iti ng
- feeling nauseous from movement
- feeling faint

- dark circles under eyes
- nighttime wakeups
- frequent urination
- IBS symptoms
- worsening allergies
- feeling better after 6 pm

- pain in the adrenal area
- high estrogen levels
- extreme fatigue
- scalp ache
- jittery or hyper feeling
- confusion

Patients have learned that it can be quite important to rule out sluggish adrenal function before starting on desiccated thyroid or T3, or soon after we have started and notice any of the above symptoms. In fact, we find it important to rule out dysfunctional or poor adrenal function even if we haven't experienced any symptoms, yet.

Testing that may not help by one's doctor

If you mention to your doctor that you have symptoms of adrenal dysfunction, you will frequently be prescribed one of the following tests, which aren't always needed:

1. ACTH Stimulation Test, also called the Stim test:

This measures your adrenal's reaction to being stimulated by the ACTH (Adrenocorticotropic) hormone. The ACTH hormone is released by your pituitary to tell your adrenals to release certain hormones, just as the TSH is released by your pituitary to tell your thyroid to release hormones. The ACTH Stim is an excellent test to detect a problem with the ACTH, which in turn could diagnose Hypopituitarism.

But there are three problems with the Stim if you suffer from the typical primary form of adrenal fatigue by hypothyroid patients: first, the test uses a bell curve to spot abnormal cortisol levels, and it only considers abnormal function to occur in the upper and lower 2% of the curve, where you would spot Addison's disease or Cushing's syndrome. Second, the ACTH Stim measures the adrenals' ability to be "stimulated", not their ability to produce enough cortisol. So, your adrenal fatigue can occur without being in these far ends of the curve, meaning your ACTH will look normal, and the doctor typically proclaims that you have no adrenal problem. Third, the stimulation you receive is about one hundred times more potent than you're ever likely to get from your own body, thus causing a response that your body would not produce on its own.

2. Blood Serum Cortisol Test:

The one-time blood test can give you an accurate measure at the time of day your blood is drawn...about your bound/unusable cortisol. What good is that!! We need to know the amount that is free and usable!

3. 24-Hour Urine Collection Test:

This test involves pouring samples of your urine into a collection container within a 24-hour period. Generally, you will urinate into your toilet first thing in the morning as normal. After that, you'll be collecting all your urine in the special container for the next 24 hours. The results then become an average of that day's period. But an average fails to tell us when we might be too high, or too low!

4. An Overnight Metyrapone or Dexamethasone Test:

Rarely used, but worth mentioning for understanding, the Metyrapone test discerns if you have an insufficient production of cortisol or a low reserve, and ascertains your pituitary gland's ability to produce enough ACTH when your cortisol levels are low. The Dexamethasone test measures the response of the adrenal glands to ACTH. Patients are usually instructed to take the medication at bedtime with a snack, then testing occurs the next morning. Because most thyroid patients don't have this kind of adrenal fatigue, these tests may not provide the information you need.

The best way to know if you have an adrenal issue

At the beginning, we have found it wise to try a few self-tests which can be done in the comfort of your own home. The first is a set of questions to ask yourself.

DISCOVERY STEP ONE:

If you answer yes to any of these, especially two or more, you may have an adrenal problem:

1. Do you have a hard time falling asleep at night?
2. Do you wake up frequently during the night?
3. Do you wake up feeling tired/unrefreshed?
4. Do get sleepy again after waking up?
5. Do bright lights bother you more than they should?
6. Do you startle easily due to noise?
7. Do you take things too seriously/easily defensive?
8. Do you cope less well with certain people or events?
9. Does it seem to take a long time to get over stress?
10. Do you feel shaky, sweaty or nauseous when you need to eat?
11. Do you feel nauseous in the face of stress?
12. Do you seem crave salt?
13. Do you feel much better after 6 pm?

When you start answering yes to two or more, you can suspect an adrenal problem.

DISCOVERY STEP TWO:

With this step, you have three tests to choose from: a pupil, temperature and/or blood pressure test. If you only choose one, the temperature test gives excellent information for overall adrenal dysfunction.

The pupil test is actually more indicative of low aldosterone, an adrenal hormone. Doing all three gives additional information. We are indebted to Dr. James Wilson, author of *Adrenal Fatigue: The 21st Century Stress Syndrome*, for inspiring us with the aldosterone pupil test as well as the blood pressure assessment in his highly recommended book, and to Dr. Bruce Rind of *www.drrind.com* for the temperature test.

• PUPIL TEST (for aldosterone levels):

Stand in a darkened room in front of a mirror. From the side (not the front), shine a bright light like a flashlight or penlight towards your pupils and hold it for about a minute. Carefully observe your pupil. With adrenal fatigue (and particularly with low aldosterone, another adrenal hormone), your pupil will get small, but it will flutter and soon enlarge again or obviously flutter back and forth in its attempt to stay constricted. With healthy levels of aldosterone, your pupil should be able to constrict and stay small for at least a minute, *even with very minor fluctuations.* NOTE: Some patients with known adrenal fatigue can pass this test, since their aldosterone levels haven't yet been affected.

• TEMPERATURE TEST:

You can determine your adrenal status by taking your temperature three times a day, starting three hours after you wake up, and every three hours after that, to equal three temps. (If you have eaten or exercised right before it's time to take your temperature, wait 20 more minutes.) Then average them for that day. Do this for at least five days. If your averaged temperatures are fluctuating from day to day more than 0.2 - 0.3 °F or .1C, you need adrenal support.

Here are the daily average results (DATS) of a patient who had confirmed adrenal fatigue (plus poorly treated hypothyroid):

> Tuesday: 98.0°F
> Wednesday: 98.3°F
> Thursday: 97.9°F
> Friday: 98.4°F
> Saturday: 98.0°F

As you can see from the above spread, there is a difference of 0.5°F from her lowest of 97.9°F to her highest of 98.4°F, implicating adrenal dysfunction.

NOTE that also applies to Chapter 6: *The comparison of averaged daily temperatures (DATS) is also an excellent method to know if you are on enough cortisol supplementation for your needs. You will do these DATS on the 6th-10th day on Adrenal Cortex or prescription hydrocortisone. If the temps fluctuate by more than 0.2F/.1C from each other, it's a clue that you need a small raise, then on the 6th – 10th day, DATS again*

Patients have found that mercury (or liquid) thermometers are the most accurate, whereas most of the digitals are not for a variety of reasons. We leave it under your tongue long enough to get an accurate temperature, which is a least 5 - 7 minutes. Mercury thermometers can be found in online auction websites like eBay, from veterinary suppliers, and in antique stores if you are diligent.

Broda O. Barnes, the author of *Hypothyroidism: the Unsuspecting Illness*, recommended measuring your tempe-rature by placing the thermometer under your arm for 10 minutes before rising in the morning., which can be ideal for the morning basal temp. You are shooting for 97.8F to 98.2F. But he also mentioned that it's about the same as doing the thermometer orally under your tongue. **For patients, oral temperature taking is the preferred method for tracking your temps.**

• **BLOOD PRESSURE TEST (the most accurate for aldosterone):**

Take and compare two blood pressure readings—one while sitting or lying down and one while standing. First, rest for five minutes in a recumbent position (sitting or lying down) before taking the first reading. Stand up and immediately take your blood pressure again. In those with healthy adrenals, the blood pressure will rise 10 - 20 points in its push to get blood to your brain. Or at the very least, it will stay the same but the latter is more ideal. If the blood pressure is lower after standing, it's a clue that your adrenals are sluggish, especially aldosterone. The degree to which your blood pressure drops while standing is often proportionate to the degree you've got low aldosterone. We have learned that doing this test in the morning can reveal a problem more readily than doing it in the evenings, but we encourage both times of the day, as one can be normal, and the other more revealing.

NOTE: This blood pressure test is also used to find the right amount of Florinef, the manmade version of Aldosterone, for those whose aldosterone test was midrange or below with symptoms. More in Chapter 6

DISCOVERY STEP THREE
(The premier way to test your cortisol levels):

If you answer yes to some of the questions, or if the tests are suspicious, patients have found it far more beneficial to do a **24-hour cortisol saliva test** (not blood), which you can order without a prescription and do right in your own home. Here's an example of one that you can order in the US or even Canada: *https://tinyurl.com/saliva-cortisol*

Testing your saliva has to be done without being on any cortisol medication or adrenal support supplements for "up to" two weeks to give a true picture of your adrenal function. We learned that we need these supplements out of our body to test and treat what is going on naturally. I do wonder if a week off for some is enough, but have no proof.

The beauty of the saliva method is that it tests your free and available cortisol levels, which blood testing does not, only testing your bound cortisol. Plus blood testing is just done once, which is inadequate, whereas saliva does it at four key times in a 24-hour period, besides being unbound. Additionally, we have found that the results of saliva testing seem to correlate almost precisely to how we are feeling.

When doing saliva tests, it can be helpful to drink plenty of fluids the day before. And on the day of the test, keep a lemon handy to sniff to help you produce plenty of spit. It generally takes up to 20 - 30 minutes to fill a vial, we have experienced.

IMPORTANT: If on thyroid meds, swallow your NDT or T3 rather than doing them under the tongue to prevent extra residue from mixing with your saliva in the vial. We also freeze each vial, and send all four, frozen, the very next day with plenty of padding to keep the cold in as long as possible, and overnight them (which can be two days in some cases.) If you fail to use the overnight delivery, you risk having your saliva deteriorate from slow delivery, giving odd results, especially in warm months.

Specific advantages of saliva over blood test

Cortisol levels can vary during the day, so saliva will test four key times at the minimum, generally 8 am, noonish, 4 - 5 pm and bedtime, whereas a blood test is often once. And there's a bonus with saliva—you don't need a prescription, and you can do it in the comfort of your own home.

Patients have found that some doctors have little knowledge about saliva testing, or they wrongly dismiss it. Granted, we have questioned saliva results for thyroid antibodies and female hormones—they seem odd at times. But *cortisol saliva results have always seemed to correlate with our symptoms of low cortisol!* Thus, we can highly recommend it to other patients, and in turn, recommend that you take the results to your next doctor's appointment and explain the correlation between the results and how you feel.

Overall, the cost of an adrenal saliva test is reasonable. But if a person can't afford it or can't find one in his or her country, yet strongly surmises sluggish adrenals based on answers to Discovery Steps One and Two, or based on the over-reactions to low doses of desiccated thyroid, it "may" be safe to experiment with cortisol support *with your doctor's guidance*, which is outlined in the next chapter. But we make no guarantees.

> **One word of caution: high cortisol symptoms can be similar to those of low cortisol, thus the strong emphasis to do the saliva test.**

Why saliva cortisol testing is the most important test you can do

Even when you are suspicious of an adrenal problem after answering the questions in Discovery Step One, or the tests in Discovery Step Two, patients have found it totally imperative to do the saliva test. Why?

First, the symptoms of too-high cortisol can be similar to too-low cortisol, and the treatment is different.

Second, the results can reveal if someone just needs adaptogens all day (seesaw results, like high, low, high, low or vice versa), or needs Adrenal Cortex (moderately low three times in a row), or prescription hydrocortisone (very low three or more times). Or if there are two highs together and two lows together, it's adrenal cortex for the lows, and certain adaptogens for the highs, like holy basil, zinc, or phosphatidyl serine. There are others. Please work with your doctor.

Understanding your saliva results

Compare below to where people are who do NOT have a cortisol problem:

> **8 am:** *at the very top of the range to help you wake up refreshed***
>
> **11 am – noon:** *in the upper quarter, but not quite as high as the morning*
>
> **4-5 pm:** *midrange*
>
> **Bedtime:** *at the very bottom, such as 1 with a range of 1 – 4, to help you fall asleep*

****IMPORTANT NOTE:** Your morning may be different than the 8 am listed above. So it's about when you normally wake up first thing---your 'morning."

Additional adrenal-related tests to consider:

- **DHEA (which saliva testing often does)**
- **Aldosterone**
- **Potassium** (can be low to serious low aldosterone)
- **Sodium** (can be too low due to low aldosterone)

DHEA (Dehydroepiandrosterone) is secreted by the adrenal glands and is a precursor for testosterone in men and estrogen in women. It appears to have many benefits beyond those hormones. As cortisol goes up, DHEA goes down. When cortisol falls, DHEA makes a last-ditch rise..then falls. .

Aldosterone is an adrenal hormone that helps regulate your blood pressure and volume. It inhibits how much sodium is released into your urine and controls your electrolyte balance (sodium and potassium plus others). Hypothyroidism can serve to create low levels of aldosterone with low cortisol. *If you also have low aldosterone in addition to your low cortisol, symptoms will include frequent urination at night (for some, in the day),*

or increased sweating, and a craving of salt.
Potassium and Sodium levels can be affected by your aldosterone. Sodium is the first lowered result to be revealed.

Choices for adrenal treatment

The beginning of Chapter 6 will explain strategies to support *healthy* adrenals in the face of stress—herbs and vitamins and a change in lifestyle.

But when saliva results reveal mostly low cortisol, we have to supplement with cortisol, as the second part of the chapter explains. Otherwise, T3 can't get to the cells and we stay hypothyroid even with thyroid treatment. **Moderately low means the use of 50 mg adrenal cortex caps in descending doses during the day; seriously low usually requires prescription hydrocortisone, such as Cortef, we have observed.**

Several highs are brought down with supplements like Holy basil, phosphatidyl serine, or zinc. There can be others which will also help lower the highs. Lowering a nighttime high and help raise the morning, but it takes several weeks.

Why HC (hydrocortisone) may be needed

For those who find themselves with serious low cortisol across the day's saliva results, the most successful treatment is achieved through the use of a prescription cortisol called hydrocortisone (HC), we have observed in our experiences, and the most well-known brand is Cortef.

Can it be difficult to find a doctor who understands treatment with cortisol? Definitely. It's crucial to do your research, study this chapter and the next, and present your information well about the large body of hypothyroid patients who have this condition, and how it's been successfully treated for years now! At the very least, it's a good strategy to find a doctor who is open-minded enough to let you take the lead based on your knowledge, while guiding you.

Controversy

The use of cortisol supplementation has a history of overuse in too high amounts (which we don't do) with serious side effects.

That fact seems to cause a knee-jerk reaction of negativity by medical professionals about its use.

But as Jeffries stated in his book *Safe Uses of Cortisol*: *"Cortisol is a normal hormone, essential for life"*. And in this case, the treatment strategy with cortisol is with physiologic doses, not the large pharmacologic doses we once saw in the past. *Physiologic refers to doses which replace, resemble or promote normal functioning, whereas pharmacologic refers to extremely high doses.*

When cortisol in the form of hydrocortisone (HC) is used to replace what your adrenals are not providing, some information and individuals will claim that 20 mg of HC is a full replacement dose, and if you go any higher, you are risking permanent suppression of your adrenals and the HPA axis (i.e. the communication between your hypothalamus, pituitary and adrenal glands). Yet others will state that the full replacement can be much higher, such as 40 mg at the minimum. *So, the question remains: how much is too much?*

What doctors and their patients who have adrenal dysfunction have discovered is that for many, staying with a cookie-cutter, one-size-fits-all amount like 20 mg or less simply doesn't adequately get thyroid hormones to the cells, no matter what studies and research implies. Temperatures can still be unstable, adrenaline is over-produced, and symptoms of low cortisol usually still persist. 20 mg may be a physiologic (beneficial) dose for a very few, but most need to start on 25 mg (women) or 30 mg (men), then find their optimal HC amounts from 27.5 to 35 mg and occasionally higher, especially with men.

One important aspect that critics of these higher doses miss is the prevalence of digestive issues from one's hypothyroidism, whether from Hashimoto's or non-Hashi's patients. Having problems with malabsorption is not uncommon—the failure to absorb from your GI (gastrointestinal) tract, and most specifically your stomach and/or intestines. The symptoms of an absorption problem may be silent, or you may have diarrhea, bloating, gas, reflux or discomfort. Thus, to achieve the same stabilization of temperatures as someone without digestive issues, adrenal patients can need more HC (or adrenal cortex/ACE) and sea salt, plus digestive aids such as Betaine HCL or one tablespoon apple cider vinegar in water.

Another fact missed by critics is the greater biological endogenous cortisol production by men vs women, i.e. men usually need higher supplementation amounts of HC (or adrenal cortex/ACE) to combat their adrenal dysfunction.

When higher doses aren't doing the trick

Some patients will find themselves having difficulty finding their right amount of HC (or even adrenal cortex), going higher and higher yet still have unstable daily average temps (it's crucial to do your daily average temps to find the right amount!). *That usually points to low aldosterone!* Thus, it's crucial to test your blood aldosterone levels, and treat low aldosterone, before going up on HC or adrenal cortex.

A small minority need to bring their doses closer together—to 3 hours apart instead of 4. So, if you were on a dosing schedule of 8 am, noon, 4 pm, and bedtime, you may need to try can try 8 am, 11 am, 2 pm, 5 pm and close to bedtime with a tiny dose.

The span of adrenal support

For the majority of hypothyroid patients with adrenal fatigue/low cortisol, treatment is not meant to be for life or several years. But for some, it can take a few months, even a year or so before all other issues are treated (that would still be stressing the adrenals) and adrenals are strong enough to succeed in a slow wean.

Additionally, HC treatment needs to be enough to take the stress off the adrenals, to stabilize one's daily averaged temperature from day to day (.2F or less apart; .1C) to build your reserves over time, and to allow thyroid hormones to adequately make it to the cells because of better cellular glucose levels.

For those with secondary adrenal fatigue, aka low cortisol production from a pituitary or hypothalamus problem, cortisol supplementation may go on for life. But you may be able to lower your cortisol somewhat after initial treatment, say some experiences.

If you have primary adrenal fatigue and the weaning fails, the problem may lie in one of four areas:

1. *You didn't raise high enough to stabilize your average temperatures five in a row. They should all be .2F or less apart (or .1C or less apart).*
2. *You failed to test aldosterone and didn't treat low levels, or didn't treat low levels correctly.*
3. *You didn't correct all other issues before weaning that continues to stress the adrenals, such as still being hypothyroid, Lyme disease, low iron, mold exposure, infections, raging Hashimoto's, chronic inflammation from any cause, any continued life stress.*
4. *You weaned far too fast. You have to do it slowly to give the adrenals times to kick in.*

When you do wean successfully, it can be helpful to support your newly-recovered adrenal function with daily high dose vitamin C, B-vitamins, minerals and herbs, adaptogens like ashwaghanda or whatever you tolerate, plus stress-dose in the face of high stress events. If you need to stress dose more than 1-2 times a week, you were not ready to come off the HC, say many patients.

Bottom line: You're not alone if you find you can't seem to tolerate desiccated thyroid, T4/T3, or T3-only, or have issues when you try to raise your dose. The corner will be turned when you recognize the problem, and treat your cortisol issues.

ADRENAL TIDBITS

* Internal shaking can be low cortisol; hand trembling is usually high cortisol.

* Headaches can be from low or high cortisol, as well as low sodium.

* Having a good sleep schedule and avoiding most any exercise is important when treating stressed adrenals.

* Females may not have stable temperatures during ovulation.

* Menopause can make women more susceptible to adrenal stress.

* If your doctor uses the Dutch version of a saliva test, we have found the cortisol results to be very wonky and not always corresponding to patient symptoms. We don't know why it's like that.

Chapter 6

HOW TO TREAT YOUR ADRENALS
(EXCELLENT CHAPTER TO SHARE WITH YOUR DOCTOR)

A drenal health is paramount for thyroid patients, and supporting them even when they are functioning well is wise. But when the adrenals are found to be dysfunctional with too high or too levels, proper treatment is equally important.

This chapter presents two of those strategies: first for those who have healthy adrenal function, but which could use support, and second for those who find themselves with a mix of high and low cortisol, or all lows, and problems when they try to raise desiccated thyroid or T3. This would be important information to share with your doctor and use in that relationship.

Adrenal Game Plan #1: for those with healthy adrenals which need support in the face of life's stressors

If saliva lab results or symptoms do not show a serious adrenal problem, but show a see-saw cortisol effect, like low, high, low, high or vice versa...or *when you are simply undergoing chronic stress and could use support*, there are a variety of strategies patients have used to assist adrenals and keep them *strong*. This can also be helpful for women who are going through the hormonal changes of peri- menopause and early menopause.

One important note: *Patient experience has repeatedly*

shown that these strategies are not enough if saliva results prove mostly low cortisol, and as proven by a 24-hour cortisol saliva test, plus the inability to use desiccated thyroid or T3 without reactions. Adrenal Game Plan #2 will need to be discussed with your doctor and implemented.

1. Vitamin C, all Vitamin B's, herbs, etc.

Your adrenal glands, made up of two sections known as the cortex and medulla, have the highest amount of Vitamin C in your body. That may partially explain why I, as author of this book, never fell into adrenal fatigue, even though I suffered extreme and constant stress on T4-only meds. I was always taking high dose Vitamin C all those years.

Thus, it may be wise to make sure you are getting adequate amounts of this important vitamin in your diet to support the function of your adrenals. Recommended amounts vary from 1000 mg to the amount you can tolerate.

The B-vitamins are also crucial for optimal adrenal function, and it's recommended to find a good balanced B-complex formula. They should include B1 (thiamine), B2 (riboflavin), B3 (niacinamide), B5 (pantothenic acid), and B6 (pyridoxine or P5P), B12 (like methylcobalamin, adensylcobalamin, or hydroxycobalamin), with special emphasis on B5 and B6. B-vitamins are well-known for their ability to counter the effects of stress. Plus, there is evidence that diet alone is not giving us enough of our B-vitamin need.

James L. Wilson, in his excellent book *Adrenal Fatigue: the 21st Century Stress Syndrome,* also recommends adding the following to your C's and B's: Vitamin E, magnesium, calcium, trace minerals, fiber and certain herbs like the licorice root, plus Ashwagandha Root and Leaf (if you tolerate them), Korean Ginseng Root, Siberian Ginseng Root, Ginger Root, Ginkgo leaf. All of the former herbs are considered adaptogens, meaning they appear to have properties which help you cope better with stress and potentially lower high cortisol, or even out a mix of highs and lows.

Rhodiola Rosea is also a popular herb and adaptogen used to counter the effects of stress and prevent adrenal burnout.

Patients report that even one dose lowered their stress, and high cortisol.

2. Laughing and enjoying your life

Your attitude towards your life can play a unique role in the continued health of your adrenals. This can especially be true for those reading this with autoimmune Hashimoto's, but also applies to those with non-autoimmune hypothyroidism. For example, the simple pleasure of laughing is said to stimulate your adrenals in a positive way, and may increase the parasympathetic supply to the adrenals.

In fact, laughing is so healthy that it can even reverse some serious illnesses, as Norman Cousins experienced and explained in his book *Anatomy of an Illness*, which I highly recommend. I remember a stressful time in my past that I consistently and purposely watched every episode of America's Funniest Home Videos—a uniquely funny television program which gave me great joy and always some belly laughs.

Another beneficial recommendation is to *slow down* and enjoy your life. No adrenals enjoy a body that goes-and-goes- as if there's no end to the going. What adrenals do love are those times each day that you stop and smell the roses. The roses can include anything that is relaxing and enjoyable. Even meditation and yoga can promote an inner joy.

This strategy can also mean to change the stressors in your life, or at the least, change the way you deal with them. Your adrenals appreciate an attitude of either *"I'm going to remove this particular stress from my life"*, or *"I'm going to accept what I can't change, and find joy around it."*

If you take your breathing for granted, don't. Take purposeful moments to take in a deep breath, hold, and release, which can break that cycle of stressful coping. In fact, do it right now and notice a renewed feeling of calm.

3. Sleeping and rest

Your body has a beneficial natural rhythm, with your cortisol at its highest in the morning to help you wake up and get going, to the lowest in the late evening to help you fall asleep.

So, the worst thing you can do to your adrenals over time is ignore your body's strong hints in the evening to go to bed. Carla explained:

> *I must have my Dad's genes, because I simply hated to go to bed at night. I resented putting down my sewing simply because my body wanted to sleep. So I fought it regularly, not going to bed until 2 am. But I noticed that I became more and more tired during the day, and I felt stressed. So I finally decided to give in to my body, and go to bed when it was telling me to, which seemed to be by 11 pm. Yeah, I resented it at first, but I then started to feel better. And to make up for going to bed on time, I found myself with better mornings to get back to my sewing.*

4. Eating frequent small meals with wise food choices

As much as supplements can be beneficial, there is no substitution for what you receive in real food, such as quality protein, vegetables, whole grains rather than refined and in moderation (for non-Hashi's patients), healthy fats and oils, and low glycemic fruits like berries. Food, especially raw foods, give us the most natural form of vitamins and minerals, fiber and phytonutrients. Phytonutrients are those compounds which help fight cancer and promote good health, including the carotenoids (that which makes a fruit or vegetable colorful, such as carrots), isoflavones (found in peanuts), or flavonoids (the red color of fruits). Flavonoids are also found in teas, but unfortunately, so is more fluoride.

On the other side of the coin, certain foods act as stimulants in some individuals, and your adrenals react. Those foods can include excess sugar, simple carbohydrates, and definitely excess caffeine. Additionally, excess sugar and carbohydrates can lead to insulin resistance due to excess insulin, and more stress on the adrenals. And again, foods like these can be bad for our Hashimoto's readers. Read the book *Hashimoto's: Taming the Beast* for info on foods from patients.

Another good strategy with the food you eat is to choose

several small meals rather than two or three large ones. This helps to keep your blood sugar levels steady and is less stress on your adrenals, as is adding good protein to each meal.

5. Keeping exercise beneficial rather than over-stimulating

The more intense your exercise routine, the more taxing on your adrenals, i.e. more ACTH is released putting demand on your already stressed adrenals. Thus, light exercise can be more beneficial, especially in times of stress.

As much as we hear or read to curtail our salt intake, healthy adrenal function thrives on salt, since cells require sodium to function optimally. But the salt of choice is unrefined sea salt, since it has a complement of absorbable trace minerals not found in table salt. This includes potassium, which helps hold water in your cells, and magnesium, which is a basic building block for adrenal hormones and supports its function.

Since unrefined sea salt is lacking in iodine, some patients feel you might want to consider adding a small amount of iodine back into your diet, via Iodoral or Lugols iodine.

For peace of mind, check your blood pressure occasionally when using sea salt, though you may find that unrefined sea salt causes no blood pressure issues. It's individual.

6. Quality over-the-counter adrenal support

Direct support of your adrenals in the face of chronic stress can be found with good OTC (over-the-counter) adrenal support supplements from your local health food store. Many of those products contain raw adrenal glandular, which is helpful. But you do have to be careful of the adrenaline in the raw adrenal glandular if you already have an excess.

Another alternative to support your adrenals in the face of life's stressors are adaptogen herbs, which has been used for a years in Chinese and Ayurvedic healing methods. Even better would be to explore *combination adaptogen products*, and taking them more than once a day. Countering chronic stress on healthy adrenals is not just once a day, we have learned.

Here are a few adaptogens, and be sure and research to see

Morning: **7.4** *(3.7-9.5)* LOW (should be close to top i.e. 9.5 or so)
Noon: **2** *(1.2-3)* LOW (should be upper quarter, lower part)
Late afternoon **1** *(.06-1.9)* LOW (should be midrange)
Bedtime **2** *(1-4)* (should always be at the bottom, so is high)

A typical starting dose of ACE for women (50 mg capsules) is 3,2,1,1, meaning three first thing in the morning, two about four hours later, one about four hours after that, and the final one in the early evening. For men, starting doses are 4,3,2,1 with the same schedule.

> *Food needs to be in the stomach with cortisol supplements to prevent nausea or stomach upset, patients have learned the hard way.*

Then, Daily Average Temps (DATS) are done on the 6th-10th day of supplementation, which is explained in Discovery Step Two in Chapter 5. We are seeing if all five averages are no more than .2F or less apart/.1C or less. If not, women raise to 4,3,2,1 and men to 5,4,3,2 of the 50 mg capsules, then do the same DATS on the 6th-10th day. For most, these raises end up being enough and giving stable averages if the starting dose does not, meaning all pairs within the five are .2F or less/.1C or less. If still not getting steady averages, it's now very important to test aldosterone via a blood test. Low aldosterone has caused us to go too high with cortisol and have unstable averages. More about aldosterone in upcoming pages, too.

> *ACE users: Please continue reading, even if the information is about very low cortisol and the use of hydrocortisone (HC). I also mention ACE if certain information also applies to ACE.*

B. When saliva results reveal _very low cortisol_

When saliva cortisol results are very low, especially three times a day, *and Addison's disease has been ruled out by one's doctor (a disease-caused very low cortisol),* it often becomes necessary to use the strength of prescription oral hydrocortisone (HC). Here's an example of **very low cortisol** from a different facility than what I showed before. The goal in the ranges still apply:

Morning: **8.8** *(6-42)* LOW (should be close to top)
Noon: **3.4** *(2-11)* LOW (should be upper quarter, lower part)
Late afternoon: **3.9** *(2-19)* LOW (should be midrange)
Bedtime: **3** *(1-8)* HIGH (should be at the bottom, so is high)

Using prescription hydrocortisone (HC): This is a stronger version of cortisol to talk to your doctor about when saliva cortisol is quite low, three or more times. The most common brand name is Cortef, but there are other names by different pharmaceuticals. It's in a bio-identical pill form and is a rapidly absorbed, man-made form of cortisol. It usually comes in amounts of 5 mg, 10 mg and 20 mg. If less is needed, then comes a handy-dandy pill cutter. Fillers can vary between brands and years, so read label if there is any concern.

The dose amount that has repeatedly shown to work best for most patients (after raising from a starting dose), i.e. optimal, will range from 25 - 35 mg of cortisol, which according to Dr. William McK. Jeffries in his book *Safe Uses of Cortisol* 'takes the strain off of the residual adrenal tissue and provides for more functional reserve in times of stress'. It's also called a "physiologic" dose of cortisol, rather than the high "pharmacologic" doses with their overriding side-effects.

A small percentage of patients may have digestive issues which causes poor absorption of what enters the stomach due to low stomach acid, so they end up higher, such as 35 - 45 mg (the latter more about men), but it's uncommon. Most are in the former category of 25-35.

Our optimal amount of HC is meant to be multi-dosed to better match the normal rhythm of our natural secretion. Examples under the heading *Starting Cortisol Amounts*.

In his paper titled *Suggestions for an Approach to the Management of Thyroid Deficiency*, UK private practitioner Dr. Barry Durrant-Peatfield recommended 20mg and up to 40 mg of cortisol to stop the symptoms of low cortisol. *But we have found that 20mg is going to underdose most of us if we need HC, i.e. it's not enough to meet our daily cortisol needs. Thus we start having problems.*

When seriously low cortisol is proven by the results of a 24-

hour cortisol saliva test, many patients find that starting on approximately **25 mg for women**, and **30 mg for men**, multi-dosed, can be helpful starting dose, as it's much closer to what their optimal amount will end up being, thus no problems. Then comes doing the Daily Average Temps (DATS) on the 6th – 10th days, and comparing them to each other to see if a small raise is needed to meet daily needs, or not.

When all of the five averages are .2F or less apart from each other (.1C or less), patients are now optimal on cortisol. Desiccated thyroid, or T3-only, can now be raised to find one's optimal dose there, too, without problems.

NOTE TO MEN: Since men secrete more cortisol than women, they often need more cortisol support. For example, where a female may end up needing 25-30ish mg of cortisol in order for thyroid hormones to fully reach the cells and temperatures stabilize, a male may need 35–40ish mg. Optimal amounts are figured out via doing and comparing the DATS. It's individual, but just as with women, you will know when your daily averaged temps stop fluctuating more than 0.2F, or .1C, from each other ((Discovery Step Two/Chapter 5).

Starting cortisol amounts: (a major change from previous editions)

When patients and curious doctors were first learning about cortisol dosing, there was an emphasis on *slowly raising* to 20 mg (which ended up being too little) and dosing 4 times a day to better replicate what the adrenals would be doing. This slow ramp up was not only in Dr. Barry Peatfield's book *(Your Thyroid and How to Keep it Healthy, Ch. 8, pg 122)*, but adrenal patients supported the slow ramp up, as well.

But it was a miserable experience to start low and go up slowly!! Slow ramping up caused very uncomfortable adrenaline surges and a shutting down of the HPA axis (hypothalamus-pituitary-adrenals) even more in response to exogenous cortisol. Some patients would freak out, thinking they were doing something wrong.

Eventually by researching/talking to each other, patients and some wise doctors came to the conclusion that "starting on" 25 mg minimum for women/30 mg for men works far better.

> *It is a disaster if we start on cortisol with a high free T3
> (usually caused by low cortisol and pooling of T3). That
> T3 rushes into the cells when cortisol is given, causing
> miserable hyper-like symptoms. Patients learned the hard
> way to lower the high pooled free T3 before starting!*

*Starting on 25 mg (for most **women** with seriously low
cortisol)*
>   10 mg first thing in the morning
>   7.5 mg four hours later
>   5 mg four hours later
>   2.5 mg   3-4 hours later (three if nighttime is stupid high)

*Starting on 30 mgs (for most **men** with seriously low
cortisol)*
>   12 mg first thing in the morning
>   10 mg four hours later
>   5 mg four hours later
>   2.5 mg   3-4 hours later (three if nighttime is stupid high)

The 4-hour dosing spread (for HC or ACE) is important for
three reasons:
1) It provides a steadier dose of cortisol since it falls
   approximately 50% (its half-life) within 1½ hours.
2) No dose is so high that it turns off our own production.
3) It better replicates your own cortisol rhythm--most cortisol
   in morning, subsequently smaller amounts during the day.

Some may need to space the doses every three hours rather
than four if they find themselves flagging before the next dose.
Others may need to add a small interim dose for about a few
months, which is easy to drop later. We figure that out if you
find ourselves flagging before the next dose.

Maximum individual dose in morning

By trial and error, wise doctors and adrenal patients
discovered that going *no higher* than 10 mg in the morning for

women, or 12 mg for men, is important, since higher doses can shut down our natural release of ACTH too much. ACTH is the hormone secreted from the pituitary gland meant to tell our adrenals to release cortisol.

Nighttime dose

Since many adrenal patients can find themselves with low blood sugar (hypoglycemia) during the night from their low cortisol, some have found that taking a small dose of hydrocortisone *(or ACE if you are on that for moderate lows)* can be needed right at bedtime to prevent the glucose lows during the night. You also want to be sure and take it with food to prevent stomach lining problems.

Taking our final dose right before we lay down results in a slower breakdown and release during the night. Dosing with 2.5mg HC at bedtime is common. Or if waking up still occurs, 5 mg at bedtime has worked for some patients. It's individual. If not tolerated, it's moved back into an earlier dose.

Men and HC dosing

Since males will usually need more HC than females, here's an example dosing schedule for a man who noticed his DATS showed a need for 37.5 mg HC (most don't need that much) and his higher metabolism dictated a 3-hour schedule (not all men will need to do this). It resembles one's circadian rhythm with highest in the morning and lowest at bedtime, and is three hours apart. If 40 mg was needed, the bedtime dose could be 5 mg, for example.

> 8 am (or upon your waking time): 10 mg
> 11 am: 7.5 mg
> 2 pm: 7.5
> 5 pm: 5 mg
> 8 pm: 5 mg
> Bedtime: 2.5

Finding the right amount of HC (also ACE)

Once a patient holds their starting dose of HC, or a raise, for at least five days, we found the importance of doing our Daily

Average Temperatures (DATS) on days 6-10 as explained in Chapter Five, Discovery Step Two. It's the steadiness of the daily averaged temperatures that will tell you if you are on the right physiologic amount for your needs. Too low or too high levels cause daily average temp instability, or averages more than .2F/.1C apart.

Once stable averages are achieved (and low aldosterone is treated if it was low), we can now raise our NDT, T4/T3 or T3-only until we have optimal frees.

How to know if we are on too much HC? Watch for these symptoms: excessive sweating, a larger increase in weight, easy bruising, weakness, facial redness or roundness, fluid retention, hump on back or even mood swings. An excess amount can also weaken our immune system, resulting in an increase in illnesses.

Why you can't use saliva testing while on HC

Unfortunately, even if some doctors try it, we found we cannot use another saliva test to ascertain if we are on the right amount. The manual addition of cortisol, with its highs after dosing, then lows from its short life, skews the results. The most accurate way to know when you are on enough is via comparing the daily averaged Temperatures. (See Chapter 5/Discovery Step 2/Temperature Test.)

About pooling of T3

If we discover low cortisol and there's a high FT3 with continued hypothyroid symptoms (pooling), we have to lower our thyroid med to lower that free T3. This will prevent the uncomfortable adrenaline/hyper surge caused by the movement of the pooled thyroid hormones rushing into the cells once we take cortisol. It can feel quite uncomfortable with extreme anxiety, racing heart, and/or other assaulting adrenaline symptoms that can last for days. If this happens, even after decreasing desiccated thyroid, doctors have guided their patients to stop desiccated thyroid or T3 completely for a day or two, then either slowly raise back up, or even better, get on straight T3 only since most will tend to have too much RT3.

Why T3-only may be better with HC (also ACE)

Unfortunately for many adrenal patients, having high cortisol levels (or low iron) can cause a build-up of Reverse T3 (RT3-the inactive hormone) from T4, which in turn, lowers your FT3 levels, making your situation worse. This is a good reason to always test one's RT3. It's too high when it's getting above the bottom two numbers of any range. Third from the bottom is a borderline number between good levels and rising levels.

One way to stop the excess RT3 production is to remove T4 from the equation, which desiccated thyroid has, too, and to start on T3-only in low doses, and raising in low amounts. It can take up to 8 weeks to fully clear excess RT3. You will also end up staying on T3-only until you have held your HC treatment for awhile, as well as corrected any issues which were causing the high RT3 in the first place (low iron, inflammation, high cortisol are the most common reasons). A few feel they may need to stay on T3 for life.

Raising thyroid while on HC (or with ACE)

After the starting dose, raising one's HC in small amounts to find steady daily average temps (DATS) is a good time to start raising one's thyroid medication, say many patients who have walked the path. If one's adrenal fatigue is severe, there may be a need to stress-dose with an extra amount of HC (or ACE) with each raise, such as 2.5 for a few days, or wait for stabilized daily averaged temps before raising.

How to avoid stomach problems with HC (also applies to ACE)

As a precaution, patients have learned to take HC with food to protect the stomach lining, which includes the bedtime dose. Some patients report nausea or stomach upsets when taking hydrocortisone without food.

Very rarely, some patients will have a hard time tolerating HC, even with food. The clue is having a reaction within an hour after taking HC. The potential solution is to cut the dose in half, taking the smallest amount you can, and raising much slower. Hydrocortisone cream rubbed into your skin, rotating the areas, is another method.

You can also take HC sublingually, but will need to watch for potential signs of thrush, which would be candida in your mouth and looks like velvety white lesions in your mouth or tongue. This doesn't happen to everyone. Some tablets are enterically coated, which will help.

The use of Hydrocortisone Cream for stomach difficulties (also ACE)

If the use of oral HC was simply too hard on one's stomach lining, even with food, one can explore the use of 1% HC cream in the treatment of their low cortisol issues. It can also give you peace of mind to keep in your pocket or purse in case you forget your HC tablets. The 1% hydrocortisone cream contains 10 mg HC per ¼ tsp. A dosing syringe can be helpful and can be found at your local pharmacy. Find the measurement for 1 ml or 1 CC on the syringe, which will also equal 10 mg HC.

Warning: it's important to rotate the places you put it on your skin, since long-term use is known to thin skin.

Interesting note: *one patient who had problems with HC hurting her stomach discovered that taking Slippery Elm Bark helped her tolerate the HC in her stomach.*

When just our morning is low (sometimes with low noon)

Sometimes, one's saliva results will simply show slightly lower levels of cortisol in the morning only, or both morning and noon i.e. your adrenals are showing very minor fatigue. If you do not have high blood pressure (which it can exacerbate) and are not on diuretics, licorice root with its Glycyrrhizic acid is a natural support of your adrenal glands since it slows and can inhibit the breakdown of cortisol in your liver.

Recommended amounts of this herb are based on your response, or around 300 - 500 mg per day. Some recommend up to 900 mg a day. Since there are no studies showing the safety of licorice root after 6 weeks, some may choose to do a two-week break and use a different support. It's not recommended if you are pregnant, have kidney or heart disease, or diabetes.

*A few patients report a pounding heart and headaches while on licorice root, even though blood pressure did not rise. Others do fine. You may **not** want to be on it long-term.*

Licorice root can be used with HC in some situations for its mineral corticoid effects, and can be helpful when you are weaning off HC.

> *Licorice root can tank potassium, so it's important to take potassium. One cup of tomato juice can contain approx. 450-500 mg of potassium.*

Sandy, who found herself with symptoms of adrenal fatigue, but couldn't afford the saliva test, states:

> *I knew I had an adrenal problem, because I had a terrible time coping when my children needed this or that, and I'd get nauseous at the drop of a hat. I also found myself shaking when I had to discipline my children. I was a single mom, too, and finances were tight. I heard about licorice root and got it. And I want to report that it made a difference in my abilities to cope. I did have to move to cortisol, but I was very impressed with what the licorice root did for me at the beginning.*

When we have high nighttime cortisol

Many adrenally-challenged patients can find themselves with high cortisol at bedtime, which promotes low cortisol in the morning or during the day (another important reason to not rely on a one-time blood cortisol test, and instead use the 24-hour cortisol saliva test). The main symptoms of high nighttime cortisol is difficulty falling asleep, or waking up the next 1-2 hours. Some don't have symptoms at all, but saliva testing proves it! If you find yourself in this boat, here are supplements that patients have found to be successful in countering the high bedtime cortisol level, one hour before you want to go to sleep.

Important to note that unlike bad information being taught in some internet or Facebook groups, you do NOT need massive amounts of any of these. That will simply stress the liver over time.

1. Phosphatidylserine, aka PS: Phosphatidyl Serine (PS) is a fatty acid found in your immune cells and muscle tissue, but is also prevalent in your brain cells. It's actually promoted as a benefit for brain improvement, such as enhancing your memory, concentration, alertness and mood, besides cell repair and improving your immune function.

But thyroid patients with high nighttime cortisol found that 300-1000 mg PS helps lower high cortisol from 30% to 70% according to different literature. PS appears to work by regulating the HPA (hypothalamus/pituitary/adrenals) axis.

When we shop for PS, we are looking for the *Phosphatidyl Serine with no complex.* Phosphatidyl Complex has made some patients feel spacey in the morning. You can also find PS in a cream to be rubbed on the skin, bypassing digestion. Seriphos is another good one.

2. Zinc: Studies report that zinc, whether doses of 25, 37.5 or 50 mg, lowers cortisol significantly even 4 hours after the dose taken. Just be sure to have food in your stomach when taking it at bedtime.[17] If copper is high, zinc can start detoxing it.

3. Holy Basil: Many studies show that this herb has proven cortisol-lowering properties. It may even help with regulating your blood sugar levels, as well as being an antioxidant. Many take 2 capsules before bed, occasionally 3 if cortisol is super high. If you have sensitivities to the Lamiaceae mint family, this is not for you.

4. Zizyphus: This popular herb, also called Jujube, is used in Chinese medicine and known for its good sedative qualities in the treatment of insomnia. Because of this sedation, it could help lower high cortisol. It's often used in combination with magnolia extracts, which may have a direct correlation in lowering cortisol.

5. Relora: This is an herbal supplement containing extracts

---

[17] https://www.ncbi.nlm.nih.gov/pubmed/1702662

of philodendron and magnolia. It has been shown to lower high cortisol levels by attaching to your cortisol receptors, which the body takes to mean it doesn't need to produce more cortisol.

Our goal with cortisol supplementation
(whether the stronger HC for very low cortisol, or ACE for moderately low)

As a thyroid patient with adrenal dysfunction, your ultimate goal with dosing is to find the least and correct amount of cortisol for your needs. For women, that appears to be around 25 - 30 mg, give or take; for men, higher. Cortisol is multi-dosed approximately four times a day with the highest dose (10 mg for women, 12 mg for men) first thing in the morning. Your optimal amount of HC, as found by doing the Daily Average Temps (Chapter 5 under Discovery Step Two), will also resolve other low-cortisol symptoms, halt the anxiety-producing adrenaline surges, and give your adrenals the rest they desperately need.

Note: if you keep raising HC higher and higher and never find stability in your Daily Average Temps, that can point to low aldosterone, which you will need to test. More on Aldosterone coming.

As far as correct doses of HC, Dr. Peatfield in the UK has mentioned that some are occasionally up to 40 mg or higher, though the latter amount may be due to poor absorption issues. It's never recommended to go higher than your needs, as revealed by DATS, to accomplish all the above. If you do go too high, and hold that high amount too long, you can risk suppression of your adrenals and immune system. Additionally, lowering high amounts of HC can be quite miserable, even if eventually successful.

Once we have achieved both goals—enough HC to stabilize your temperatures (found by doing one's Daily Average Temps) and optimal treatment of your hypothyroidism—it takes great stress off of our adrenals. Additionally, treating low cortisol, optimizing our thyroid treatment, and treating low iron can help rebalance sex hormones in some individuals; others may need to treat their sex hormone imbalances directly.

Raising HC

Fast is not in the dictionary for adrenal treatment. We have noted that it can take several days for the effects of the cortisol to be apparent, especially the leveling out of your average temperatures (using Daily Average Temps) and stopping the adrenaline surges that can happen on the lower, non-optimal doses. Paying attention brings the best information and results, as well as changing one thing at a time.

> Note: *giving ourselves too much cortisol can also cause unstable temperatures. That's why patients only go up by 2.5mg HC or 1-2 of 50mg ACE), and do their Daily Average Temp comparisons five days after each raise.*

Important: While raising HC, patients have found it wise to be on some tolerable amount of thyroid hormones. Without thyroid to work with, cortisol can go too high over time, even though at first, it was the right amount.

Stress dosing with HC (also applies to ACE)

Everyday stressful events: Healthy adrenals would produce extra cortisol in times of physical or emotional stress to enable your body to cope. Knowing that fact, adrenally-challenged patients on the right amount of cortisol have realized they will need to stress dose in the face of a long-term or a single highly stressful event, a body injury, or illness like the flu or worse.

In fact, stress dosing can be extremely important for adrenal patients to prevent an adrenal crisis in the face of a stressful event. This is why patients state they keep hydrocortisone cream with them at all times when not at the house.

For those one-time events like a friend, loved one, child or boss who is in a rage, and at the first sign of a pounding heart or shakiness, a good stress dose can start at 2.5 mg, but if stress still causes issues within the half hour, another 2.5 to equal 5 mg can work.

that is a lot.

For serious illnesses like the flu: When an illness like the flu approaches, one method used by patients is to immediately add 20 mgs HC, twice daily and for three days. Then taper it down to 7.5 twice daily, then 5 mg twice daily, then back to a former dose.

Three days and up to 20 mg per day is the maximum for stress dosing in most cases, though there are occasional situations like unwanted family members during a holiday that can spell longer stress dosing.

Jeffries, in his book *Safe Uses of Cortisol* states:

> [In events of stress] *higher dosages of cortisol are required to maintain a physiologic state that would produce hypercortisolism with its well-known undesirable effects in the unstressed states. The increased secretion of adrenal hormones serves to meet an increased need during stress and tends to maintain homeostasis rather than to disturb it. The increased secretion does not cause a state of hypercorticism such as develops when the titer of these hormones is increased artificially in the absence of need. Hence, a patient with adrenal insufficiency under stress may require dosages of cortisol to maintain a physiologic state that would produce hypercortisolism with its well-known undesirable effects in the unstressed state. This higher amount can be up to double what you would normally take daily.*

Once patients stress-dosed for a few days, or the illness has started to subside, doctors guide patients to taper off the extra amounts *a little at a time*, and slowly, eventually ending up with the amount they were previously on.

> **Note:** *if we find yourself frequently stress-dosing for emotional stress, we may simply not be on enough HC with stabilized temps.*

When higher doses of HC aren't doing the trick

It's not the norm and you will be in the minority, but some

patients definitely experience that doses higher than 35 - 40 mg of HC are not helping thyroid hormones make their move from the blood, perhaps due to digestive issues, a resistance, or a problem with metabolizing HC too quickly between doses. And the higher doses increase the risk of side effects, including water retention, since HC has salt-retaining properties.

So with their doctor's guidance, they then move to a five-times stronger, longer-acting Glucocorticoid such as methyl-prednisolone with a brand name of Medrol. It's either a partial dose or a total treatment. Medrol has lower fluid-retaining properties than HC, seems to have less side effects, such as a decreased danger of high blood pressure, and less stress on your liver.

But Medrol can be much harder to dose, and it should be used only as a last resort. In conversion amounts, 1 mg of Medrol is equal to approximately 5 mg of HC. Patients who make the switch can end up on 6 mg of Medrol, spread out over the day, such as 3 mg first thing in the morning, 2 mg in the mid-afternoon, and 1 mg at bedtime.

If stress-dosing is needed on Medrol, patients use HC.

All the following apply to either HC or ACE

DHEA—to take or not take *Vic says NEVER with PCOS.*

DHEA is another stress hormone released by your adrenals and is a counter balance to your cortisol. And when cortisol gets low, so does your DHEA eventually fall. Some research claims that DHEA supplementation can further lower one's already-low cortisol levels, whereas other research shows no decline as a result of DHEA.

In groups, you'll find some patients stating they feel well on DHEA. As a result of these mixed study results and experiences, the only way to know if DHEA supplementation is lowering your cortisol is by doing temp taking as outlined in Discovery Step Two in Chapter 5.

Cortisol and weight gain

Many patients who treat their sluggish adrenals with

hydrocortisone report unwanted weight gain. There are a few reasons it can happen.

So maybe creates open to (handwritten margin note)

1. *Oral administration of HC may encourage the body to produce glucose (blood sugar), which in turn causes fat production and storage from the excess insulin.*
2. *The mineral content of HC can contribute to water gain.*
3. *The most likely reason: you need to start raising your thyroid meds as you get closer to your right amount of HC.*
4. *You may be on too much and need to talk with your doctor about slightly lowering it while still maintaining stable daily averaged temperatures.*

Whatever the cause, we find it prudent to watch our diet far more closely than before, focusing on proteins and vegetables as the main part of your daily consumption, and much less on carbohydrates. When carbohydrates are consumed, choosing those that are low glycemic is a positive decision, since low glycemic carbohydrates are digested much slower than high glycemic. Examples of low glycemic foods include high fiber grains, berries, cottage cheese, meats, most vegetables, etc.

Since Hashimoto's patients should be avoiding gluten in grains, they may need to study which low glycemic foods they can tolerate. *See Hashimoto's: Taming the Beast.* Foods for anyone to curtail or avoid are sugars, potatoes, pasta, white rice, and white flour products.

Sex Hormones

Some patients have discovered they can't wait on their optimal HC use to address their sex hormone issues with their doctors. So they start to treat those problems while working on their HC. Testosterone supplementation is one example, since HC use can lower your testosterone levels. And if you were already low, this can be a problem. Low estrogen often needs to be addressed since it can exacerbate high glucose levels, or trigger hypoglycemia (low blood sugar).

Muscle weakness

The use of cortisol, even the smallest amounts, initially can cause your testosterone levels to tank, as it can potassium. Low estrogen makes the weakness worse. This is especially a problem if you are a woman and have no ovaries or are into menopause. So you may need to talk to your doctor about testosterone and potassium supplementation for the first few weeks or months of your cortisol use. *But I don't want more!*

Problems tolerating cortisol supplementation

Most of the time, patients have found that problems with HC are actually from taking too little, or needing to dose closer together, such as every 2-3 hours, to help build low reserves.

Cortisol and blood pressure

If you have high blood pressure when you start on any cortisol treatment, it's a good choice to monitor your blood pressure during the treatment and keep in touch with your doctor as to the trends of your blood pressure. Treatment of aldosterone can also cause changes in your blood pressure.

Even if you don't have high blood pressure, monitoring blood pressure and pulse is a good idea while dosing HC. Both give you good clues about your HC dosing.

Exercising with adrenal dysfunction and cortisol supplementation

Adrenal patients have found out repeatedly that almost *any form of moderate to intense exercise has been unhealthy for their challenged adrenals.* Why? To the degree that you exercise, to the same degree demand is put on your adrenals. That can be a hard message to hear when some individuals have valued their exercise routine. Instead, rest and more rest can be the most recommended response to assist in adrenal treatment and stabilization. I tell adrenal patients to look at it like taking a different path in your life—a healthy path that is extremely important.

Waking up during the night

High bedtime cortisol causes frequent waking up, especially 1-2 hours after going to bed. But low nighttime cortisol also causes many patients to wake up in the middle of the night from the adrenaline rush and hypoglycemia, aka low blood sugar. The solution is having the last dose of your total daily amount of HC at bedtime, such as 2.5 with food is tried first. If waking up continues, those patients move that up to 5 mg.

Another strategy used by patients who know they are waking up from low cortisol is to immediately take two Adrenal Cortex when they wake up.

If confused what is going on at night, there are some labs which offer six saliva testing times—two of those are during the nighttime. This is one called Sabre, an affiliated link: *https://www.directlabs.com/sttm/OrderTests.aspx*

Salt and adrenals

As mentioned at the beginning of this chapter for continued support of already-healthy adrenals, salt is also a necessary supplement to treat flagging adrenals (if blood pressure isn't high). It isn't coincidental that adrenal dysfunction, especially in the presence of low aldosterone, another adrenal hormone, causes you to crave salt. When your adrenals become sluggish and aldosterone goes low, salt can be released from your body via your urine and you become sodium deficient. And since the cells in your body require sodium to function optimally, it's especially important to give sodium back to yourself.

The salt of choice is unrefined sea salt, since it has a complement of absorbable trace minerals not found in table salt, as well as lacking excess aluminum. Sea salt also includes potassium, even if in minute amounts, plus magnesium, which is a basic building block for adrenal hormones and supports its function. You can add unrefined sea salt to a liquid such as water or orange juice (for added potassium), but be careful with orange juice if you tend to have blood sugar issues. Recommended amounts of sea salt are approximately ½ tsp, and up to twice a day.

Since unrefined sea salt is lacking in iodine, some patients will add iodine via Iodoral or Lugols iodine. For peace of mind, we check our blood pressure occasionally when using sea salt. We also keep potassium up.

Low aldosterone

Turns out that quite a few adrenal patients, at least 50% with low cortisol (a subjective observation) also have an aldosterone problem. Aldosterone, a mineralocorticoid hormone, helps regulate levels of sodium and potassium in your body when your adrenals are healthy—i.e. it helps you retain needed salt, which helps control your blood pressure and the distribution of fluids in the body. In turn, it contributes to balance of the electrolytes in your blood like calcium and magnesium, and helps prevent potassium from rising too high.

When aldosterone gets too high, especially in the face of chronic stress, your blood pressure also gets too high and your potassium levels can go too low. You can have muscle cramps, muscles weakness, and numbness or tingling in your extremities. Even scarier, research has shown that chronically high aldosterone can shorten one's life, perhaps due to higher blood pressure.

When aldosterone gets too low, which is the most common situation for adrenal fatigue patients, your kidneys will excrete too much salt, and it can lead to low blood pressure, low blood volume, a high pulse, and/or palpitations, dizziness and or light-headedness when you stand, fatigue, and for some, a craving for those salty potato chips in your cupboard.

Symptoms of low aldosterone can also include frequent urination, sweating, and a feeling of thirst, plus feeling hot. When is serum sodium too low? *In a range of 135-145, 135-139 is too low.*

Many patients with low sodium levels have chosen to treat the symptoms of low aldosterone with supplemental sea salt in water and sipped on all day. Some start on ¼ tsp, taken twice a day to equal ½ tsp total. Some move to ½ tsp twice day. It's individual.

But...a large body of research reveals that the more sodium you give yourself, the more your aldosterone will fall, as well as your angiotensin II, a peptide hormone which works with aldosterone to find the right balance of sodium and potassium. i.e. too high levels of sodium will cause further lowering of your already-low aldosterone, which could still lower your sodium again. And the more sodium you ingest, the thirstier you can be. It's a balancing act each person has to figure out. That's why the recommendation stops at ½ tsp twice a day.

Additionally, when the adrenals are not making aldosterone, our renin, a hormone from the kidneys, increases. (If the renin is low, you could have a pituitary problem.)

Testing aldosterone

The most important thing to know about testing your serum aldosterone is that it's a must, since both low and high aldosterone can have similar symptoms in some. The day before your test, you'll want to avoid salt in any form, whether avoiding the salt shaker, sodas, French fries, cottage cheese, pizza or any high salt foods. Fast after you go to bed. Note that Motrin, as well as beta blockers, steroids and diuretics, can affect your result.

The testing is best done in the morning and after you've been moving around for the morning, which boosts aldosterone levels. You'll want to be sitting for the blood draw.

It's important to know that aldosterone levels can be doubled if you are pregnant, and are normally a little higher in children than in adults. For women, it's best to do the test within the first week after you start your period, since your rising progesterone levels can affect the aldosterone.

For a complete picture, ask your doctor to include your renin, as well as sodium and potassium, for testing at the same time. Low aldosterone can also be detected by low serum sodium results. You can test the latter two without a prescription and bring the results to your doctor. See Addendum D for facilities.

What have we seen that equals "low aldosterone"? Midrange or lower, as it includes clear symptoms of low aldosterone, too.

Treatment for low aldosterone

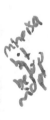

Since low aldosterone can lower potassium if it's gone on awhile, we have found that one of the first treatments a patient should consider (if labs show low potassium) is prescription slow-release potassium. Slow release prescription potassium in high amounts has helped many patients. Labs are retested every 2-3 weeks to make sure you don't go too high. Work with your doctor.

Directly for the low aldosterone, even the use of licorice root can be helpful since its glycyrrhizin mimics aldosterone in affect. But watch your blood pressure, say patients, which licorice root can raise. It can also lower that potassium. So taking higher amounts of potassium is a must.

If raising potassium and using licorice root hasn't helped, the prescription medication of choice for low aldosterone is fludrocortisone acetate, aka **Florinef**. Talk to your doctor about starting with a quarter of the 100 mcg pill rather than starting on the full pill, since it's very potent. It's also recommended to take your Florinef with a small amount sea salt mixed in water, but it's not required.

With each dose of Florinef, one is watching whether the BP test has improved (Standing BP rises above the seated BP), as shown in Chapter 5, Discovery Step Two. If not, patients raise a quarter pill every 7-10 days depending on the tests. The goal is to get to the full pill, or until blood pressure is normal and symptoms of low aldosterone disappear. It's not uncommon to need 1-2 pills, even 2 pills total, before getting the blood pressure to rise upon standing as compared to when sitting.

When keeping track of your blood pressure, make sure your arm is resting perpendicular to your body, not downward—the latter a mistake that many nurses and doctors make.

One way to know we are on too much Florinef is by high blood pressure, fluid retention and/or pressure headaches. Also, even when you are on the right amount of Florinef, it can lower serum potassium levels as a side effect, so it's crucial to supplement with potassium, say many patients and doctors, and keep track of potassium labs. Note that one cup of tomato juice is roughly equivalent to 450-500 mg potassium. Check your label.

It's also important to note that some patients who are already on HC or ACE, may have to lower either to compensate for the glucocorticoid potency within Florinef. Later, when one feels ready to wean off HC or ACE, patient experience has shown that it's better to stay on Florinef a little longer before weaning off Florinef.

If a patient finds Florinef to have uncomfortable side effects like dizziness or nausea (not common), and they need to come off of it, patients usually end up raising their HC a tad and increasing sea salt consumption. Talk to your doctor.

How long we will need to be on HC (or ACE)

The bottom line is: "when we have fully treated anything that continues to stress the adrenals". i.e. we need:

- "optimal" on thyroid meds, not just "on them"
- optimal levels of iron/B12/vitamin D and any other nutrients
- fully treated Lyme or reactivated EBV (Epstein Barr virus)
- free from mold exposure and/or treated it
- Hashimoto's antibodies down
- treatment of any other autoimmune issues
- successful lowering of chronic inflammation
- avoids or moderates any chronic stress
- good food with good nutrients
- avoids any triggering foods

After we achieve all the above, patients found they can start a very slow wean of their cortisol supplementation to allow their adrenals to kick in.

Remember: if you are the minority with adrenal fatigue due to Hypopituitary, a secondary cause of your adrenal fatigue, you may need to be on HC the rest of your life. Work with your doctor on this.

Letting others know of our HC or ACE use

We as patients feel it's important to use an ID bracelet or information in our wallet about our daily amount of cortisol supplementation, as well as the name of our doctor and phone number. We can also inform close family members or friends what we are doing. We also find it prudent to keep extra hydrocortisone pills or cream with us when we are expected to be gone from the house for several hours. The worst thing we want to do, in your attempt to have better health and de- stress our adrenals, is to forget a dose, or not have what we need when it's time.

Weaning slowly is the key

Patients and their doctors have learned that the beginning of a successful wean means to cut off only 2.5 mg per 2-3 weeks at the minimum. Remember, by weaning, your rested adrenals are suddenly being encouraged to make up the slack. Let them get the message with ease. You can start by weaning off the latest dose, and then slowly move upwards in the day, or whatever time seems to work best for you.

We have discovered the importance of timing the wean to occur during the least stressful time of your daily life. This means avoiding holidays, stressful events or busy times of the year. If during your weaning process you encounter stress, you may have to stress dose as mentioned above. It will slow down the wean, but it will also prevent further stress on your adrenals.

When we feel ready to wean, consider it a *huge no-no* to stop cortisol supplementation suddenly. This can create an adrenal crisis – a life-threatening situation where your body is suddenly without the crucial cortisol. Symptoms include low blood pressure and weakness, headache or nausea, shaking or confusion, a rapid heart rate, excess fatigue, or sweating.

Failures in weaning

When weaning is difficult, it usually means s patient didn't achieve successful treatment of all the issues listed previously.

Post-weaning strategies to keep the success (HC or ACE)

Once you have successfully weaned off your cortisol, there are important follow-up strategies to promote continued success, we have learned. One is to continue over-the-counter adrenal support for a few months, especially in response to stress. Supplementing with vitamin C, B-vitamins, and other anti-stress vitamins, herbs and minerals can also be beneficial. Removing stressors in your life is important. Comparing your daily averaged temperatures can continue to be a monitor as to your adrenal recovery progress.

Perry, a thyroid and adrenal patient, developed the following tips for weaning:

1. For some amount of time after weaning (6 months? We don't know yet), your adrenals will be weak, and you will need to support them whenever stress re-enters your life.

2. The sooner you recognize the stress and respond with adrenal support, the more likely you are to avoid a major crash.

3. If you know something stressful is coming, you should begin supporting your adrenals before it happens. How much before depends on when this future event begins to occupy your mind (and cause stress).

4. Some early signs to look for are: a desire to snack continually; a tendency to "withdraw" from friends, family, and favorite activities; an exaggerated startle reflex; a tendency to get flustered by normal events like telephone calls; overreacting to the words or actions of others; a return of any of the symptoms you experienced the first time you needed adrenal support.

5. Adrenal support after recovery for periods of less than one week can be discontinued abruptly. If support is used for one week or longer, it should be tapered off at the same rate as you originally weaned. For hydrocortisone, a good rate seems to be reducing by 2.5 mg every 2 - 3 weeks.

6. Some events to watch out for and are nearly always stressful are: vacations; family visits; holidays; dental work; colds, flu, and other illness.

7. Don't consider going back on adrenal support as a defeat. Using adrenal support as needed during the recovery period will help you ultimately be successful in recovering full adrenal function.

High cortisol

What if, unlike all the latter information, you find yourself with high cortisol three or four times on a saliva test? As author of this book, this is exactly what happened to me. And if I didn't do something quickly, I was destined to fall into the more serious stages where the adrenals can't keep up and cortisol becomes low.

My own high cortisol was due to a long-term use of *too-high doses* of topical progesterone to counter high estrogen. Once I figured it out, I stopped the supplementation. Within a few days, strong signs of progesterone overuse, similar to estrogen dominance symptoms, stopped. But I still had weeks of treatment to lower my high cortisol, and which included the committed use of PS, as mentioned above. Today, I favor Holy Basil.

High cortisol can go on for awhile before you realize it's happening. When it finally rears its ugly head, you can have similar symptoms to low cortisol: easy fatigue, nausea in the face of stress, shakiness, lowered temperature, depression, achiness, etc. You will also tend to have rising or high blood pressure. Additionally, because high cortisol makes conversion of T4 to T3 difficult, you end up having far too much T4 and a conversion to Reverse T3—the latter which will serve to block regular T3 from making it to your cells.

The only way to accurately know you have high cortisol is to do the 24-hour saliva cortisol test. *http://www.tinyurl/saliva-cortisol* The reasons you may have high cortisol are varied: chronic emotional stress, chronic health conditions, blood sugar problems, poor eating or sleeping habits, a compromised immune system, severe exhaustion, heart disease, too much weight, or like me, the use of topical progesterone. Each person has to figure out their own catalyst, and change it.

Using T3 in early morning hours to raise low morning cortisol—the CT3M method

UK Thyroid patient Paul Robinson discovered something quite fascinating—that poor adrenal function could be related to poor adrenal tissue levels of T3. And one could bring back better function by a unique way of using T3-only in the early morning hours. He states this would only work if one does not have diabetes, insulin resistance or other blood sugar regulation issues, hypopituitary or Addison's disease. The latter conditions would dictate the use of HC.

Now before you get excited about this, doing the CT3M is **not** a quick and easy alternative to ACE or HC. Some people don't like waking up that early to take their T3, then to have to fall back asleep. And there have been several who have reported it did nothing for the low afternoon. But for low morning and sometimes noon, it's been a great alternative, say patients who have tried it.

It's also important to know that you have to be precise in keeping the same schedule the majority of the time to make this work well. If you have wonky wake up times or you don't take the T3 at a consistent time, it may not work well for you

Important general points he discovered are as follows:

1. Most of the day's cortisol is made by one's adrenals in the last four hours of sleep before waking up. For example, if one naturally wakes up at 8 am, that window would be 4 - 8 am. And since adrenal cells need T3 as any cell would, giving oneself T3 in that 4-hour window would be key.

2. One's first T3 dose of the day, such as 12.5 - 20 mcg, is usually started about 1 – 1 ½ hours before one wakes up for the day, held a few weeks while watching daily blood pressure, pulse and temperature. Then it's moved up earlier by half an hour, held, and data repeated. The goal is looking for the time in that window when the adrenals seem to kick in the best, as shown by temperature, blood pressure and heart rates which return to normal. Many find that time to be in the first 1-2 hours of that 4-hour window. If good adrenal response is not found, and one was on a lower amount of T3, the process is repeated with an increase of 5 mcg.

3. If a particular time gives too much of a response, one puts the T3 later again by half an hour.

4. Better adrenal response can occur in three months if the protocol is done correctly, while other T3 doses are continued throughout the day.

Robinson underscores that one will need to be on a good B-complex, B12, Vitamin C several times daily, Vitamin D, a good chelated multi-mineral, and chelated magnesium.

If someone tries this while on HC (details below), Robinson feels it's best to try and reduce HC as much as possible, and definitely try small (2.5 mg) decreases while doing the protocol. He also feels it's important to do an ACTH Stim test to confirm that the adrenals are capable of responding to the early morning T3 doses. Finally, direct T3 is needed instead of slow-release T3. You can find his books on Amazon.

The bottom line of adrenal support

We as patients have learned that the sum and substance of adrenal support is that which is easiest yet effective. After finding out what is going on via a Cortisol Saliva test (it's NOT about guessing), and comparing our results to where patients are who don't have a cortisol problem, it can be the...

a) use of adaptogens to counter the highs and lows of early stress

b) the use of adrenal cortex for those of us with moderately low levels

c) the use of prescription cortisol for seriously low levels, where Addison's has been ruled out.

Rejuvenation of our adrenals, once fatigued, can take time and patience, following known successful methods as outlined in this chapter, as well as particular lifestyle changes away from stress. It can be slow, but the progress will be there!

ADRENAL TIDBITS

* The cortisol you take earlier in the day for low cortisol levels will eventually help drop too-high levels later in the day.

* A high heart rate can be from high cortisol, low cortisol, low sodium, low potassium, low magnesium, low iron and more.

* You won't recover from illness while on HC as fast as you would have with healthy adrenal function, say some.

* A slightly higher temperature can be from too much thyroid, too low aldosterone, or low iron.

* A certain body of patients with adrenal issues choose to switch to T3-only due to high levels of RT3.

* When supplementing with HC or even Adrenal Cortex, cortisol levels can go too high if one is not taking any thyroid to help clear the cortisol.

* Having a hard time finding stable Daily Average Temps after raising and raising cortisol again? That can point to low aldosterone. So we go back down a bit, and deal with aldosterone testing and treatment.

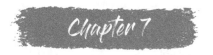

Chapter 7

THE DOCTOR CHAPTER

*For this is the great error of our day that the physicians
separate the soul from the body*

HIPPOCRATES

Many times over numerous years while on either
Synthroid or Levoxyl, I felt like a worn-out piece of
over-chewed bubble gum. And I just knew that a visit
to a doctor was the answer, no matter how far I had to drive or
how long the appointment took.

In fact, who as a thyroid patient, hasn't felt immeasurable
hope that a doctor was going to help. And why not? They've
had the most immense education and demanding training of
most any profession, including several years of internship and
residency before they even hang their shingle on the door.

So when you walk into their offices, it's like the once familiar
Allstate Insurance commercial refrain: *You know you're in good
hands.* The doctor or health professional is going to prescribe
the right pills or use the best therapy to help you turn the
corner towards better health.

*Yet, to the degree thyroid patients have had high hopes
in their highly educated and experienced doctor, to the same
degree that hope has repeatedly turned to dust too many times.*
In fact, the compelling and descriptive experience of thyroid
patients globally with their doctors ranges anywhere from
disappointing, frustrating and sad...to shabby, disrespectful,
ignorant, patronizing, pompous, close-minded and/or bordering
on malpractice.

Endocrinologist are often reported by patients as the worst, as well (even if there can be a few exceptions).

Intense, real, and extremely pitiful.

Are there doctors who are the rule to the exception? Yes. Their numbers have been growing thanks to the patient-to-patient Stop the Thyroid Madness movement that has influenced even other groups and websites. Some doctors are listening. Some doctors are open-minded. Some are treating patients with respect. We so appreciate you!

Unfortunately, though, progress is slow within the wider ranks. Stephanie, a thyroid cancer survivor who gives thanks, in part, to her use of desiccated thyroid, remembers vividly the doctor of whom she first asked about prescribing Natural Desiccated Thyroid. She had already observed the benefits it was giving other hypothyroid patients, and felt it was a right choice for her, as well. Here's what she wrote in her blog:

First, he breezes into the room and shakes my hand and exclaims "Well we had you on 0.175 mg of Synthroid and you were experiencing hyper symptoms (TSH was 0.024) and we reduced your dose to 0.150 mg but now your TSH is WAY too high so we need to bump you back up to the 0.175 mg dosage again." EXCUSE ME???? I felt bad on 0.175 mg and 0.150 mg isn't working, so let's just put you back where you felt bad and not think about options?? UGH!! I didn't say this but thought it.

This is the point where I interjected that I wanted to know where my Free T3 numbers were so I had them run. I produced my lab slip for him. I told him that I had been studying T3 and how some people don't convert T4 to T3 well. He went on and on about how it wasn't true that they had done lab tests on dead babies and had found T3 in them. I said "WHAT???". I said "Listen again–I didn't say that I didn't make T3 at all but that I could be someone who didn't convert it WELL enough to give me what I needed." He quickly changed his tune and said "Oh I know what we can do. I'll leave you on the 0.150 mg since you seem to feel well on that (never asked me how I was feeling though just assumed that since I hadn't called, I was OK) and we'll add some synthetic T3–It's called Cytomel". UGH! I swear he thinks I am an idiot and it is so patronizing! I already knew his protocol before I got to his office.

So at this point I interject with "Can I try natural desiccated thyroid?" You should have seen how fast he looked up from his paper that he was writing on. The entire time he was telling me what we were going to do he couldn't take the time to look at me prior to this. He exclaimed "ABSOLUTELY NOT." I asked "Why not?" This pushed his buttons as he physically began to shake. I got the "Because it isn't for you." So I pushed further–"Why not?" Then he gives me the canned answer (I think they get this in Endo school) "Because it isn't stable." I said "What do you mean?" I swear this man was about ready to strangle me for asking questions and questioning his authority but I pressed on. He said "Because it is from a Pig and you don't want to take pig hormones."

As Stephanie continues in her blog, the doctor proceeded to give a variety of negative and condescending explanations against pig thyroid, including she would die if she took it.

I left his office and went out to my car and cried. It is very hard to have a Dr. tell you that you will die of cancer if you take NDT–whether you believe it or not.

In the notes in her doctor's chart, he wrote the following:

Stephanie states that she would like to try NDT. I told her that this is unacceptable and I would not place her on it. She will have to see another physician if she wants to try this medication because it is animal derived and the T3 & T4 levels are not closely regulated, and cannot be independently adjusted.

It doesn't take much to imagine how Stephanie may have

felt as she was leaving this doctor's office. Feeling awful, she was now being told that what might make her feel better, was not acceptable.

The experience of patients

When you peruse most any thyroid patient group on the internet, or talk to thyroid patients one-on-one, you find that there are a myriad of common and heart-wrenching negative stories about visionless, indiscriminate pill-dispensing, medical practitioner zombies.

Additionally, most thyroid patients will state they have been harmed when they discover how ineffective T4-only really is, or the failure of the TSH lab test as the so-called "gold standard" of diagnosis and treatment. Additionally, they will state extreme harm when they find themselves with poor adrenal output as a result of both of the above.

Being harmed by one's doctor is an action polar opposite to the oath of standards and ideals that most physicians took when they were about to embark in their medical practice.

Have doctors come to see their medical school oath as nothing more than a staid, rote and meaningless ritual? Part of the original Hippocratic Oath, which some schools have grossly modified or removed, states in the original Greek:

> *To please no one will I prescribe a deadly drug nor give advice which may cause his death.*

Yet, nothing has been more deadly to thyroid patients for decades than a drug called thyroxine so exuberantly prescribed by too many doctors, and which has served to leave patient patients with some residual hypothyroid symptoms. This is equally so for the TSH lab test and its dubious "normal" range.

All you have to do is read my own story of 17 years (see Introduction), going from doctor to doctor, and not finding one who was thinking beyond his or her medical school training box to observe that perhaps thyroxine for hypothyroid was not working, or that the "normal" TSH range did not to conform to my clinical presentation! I also had to endure doctors who were dismissive, close minded, and condescending, even if well-meaning.

Aspects of my story, Stephanie's experience, and worse, can be found in millions of thyroid patients across the world. This is not a scenario that only involves a few. So now, we have to ask: *are physicians listening?*

Four crucial mistakes made by practitioners

Thyroid patients all over the world are growing in their knowledge and truth against what doctors have been doing. I now highlight four crucial and consequential mistakes that most all patients have experienced. Each mistake represents an area that needs drastic change:

1. Making the TSH lab work, or "normal" ranges, the holy grail of diagnosis.

Of all the mistakes listed, this misjudgment has been the most widespread and damaging. Put yourself in the shoes of a patient who enters his or her doctor's office with factual and obvious hypothyroid complaints of continuing poor stamina, feeling cold, gaining weight, dry skin, hair loss, rising cholesterol and/ or depression, only to be callously told that because the TSH or other lab results are within range, he or she is "normal". Thus, it's concluded that her symptoms have nothing to do with hypothyroid. So, the doctor reasons, she needs other medications to treat the 'non-thyroid' symptoms, to eat less and exercise more, or see a psychiatrist.

Hogwash!

It has occurred not only when a patient first enters the office, having no prior thyroid diagnosis, but even more maddening when the patient is T4-only, or underdosed on desiccated thyroid or T3.

The litany from patients who have experienced this schizophrenic "normal" diagnosis in the face of continuing symptoms is full of angst. "*I must be crazy!*" is the outcry of this all-too-common encounter with doctors.

LeeAnn relates the following crazy-making scenario:

I was on Synthroid for 7 years, and I was depressed. There was no depression in my biological family, I had a happy marriage, and I loved my job in the courthouse. I made a lot of appointments with doctors, and each and every one told me I had a psychological problem. Three pushed antidepressants on me, one insisted I needed to admit myself in a mental health facility at the Presbyterian Hospital, and two told me I needed to make an appointment with either a Psychiatrist or Psychologist. I fought it for a long time, then decided maybe I AM nuts and need help. It was chilling, let me tell you.

Many years and decades before thyroid lab work came into existence, doctors paid attention to symptoms and dosed by those symptoms (as well as the exclusive use of desiccated thyroid). Today, the clinically presenting symptoms and signs of hypothyroid are no less obvious than a nose on a face, yet the constellation of hypo- symptoms are routinely dismissed if ink spots on a piece of paper state otherwise. It's a one-track worship of the dubious TSH lab with its erroneous "normal" range, or the total T4 or just the free T4, without a free T3. So patients are left hanging over the alligators of their obvious hypothyroid symptoms with a doctor proclaiming *"You are normal."*

You can also have a patient on desiccated thyroid who walks into the office feeling wonderful– full of energy, lowered cholesterol, freedom from depression, thickening hair–yet because of a suppressed TSH, the patient is told to lower the desiccated thyroid, which only results in the return of previous hypothyroid symptoms.

2. Maintaining complete ignorance about desiccated thyroid

Any thyroid patient who has dared to ask about desiccated thyroid has heard every single possible *misconception* there can be from the mouths of our doctors. Because of that, you come to believe that not one doctor can think beyond his medical school training, continuing education, medical journals, or the lips of his favorite pharmaceutical rep. *It's as if the experience of patients who have successfully used desiccated thyroid, past and present, is completely invisible.*

Even worse are those patients who are citizens of countries where the use of a beneficial like desiccated thyroid or T3 is banned! Though there can be closed walls because of religious beliefs towards pork, the majority of patients who contact me about their nation's prohibition of desiccated thyroid appear to describe a misconception of the safety of the direct T3 in desiccated thyroid, or synthetic T3 itself.

The following are actual one-word descriptions made by numerous doctors to their patients about desiccated thyroid. As reported to patients by patients, they represent the ignorance that abounds among medical professionals, ranging from sublimely false to the absurdly ridiculous:

Unreliable
Unstable
Dangerous
Inconsistent
Old-fashioned
Outdated
Unconventional
Unregulated Harmful
Toxic

Isn't it interesting that the only word that we have found to be true about desiccated thyroid is that it's *old-fashioned*, just as it might be old-fashioned to wear clothes from your past that still feel good, or use vintage tools that still work well?

Patients have repeatedly experienced desiccated thyroid to be quite *reliable, safe, consistent from dose-to-dose, regulated by the USP, modern, conventional and with life- saving results* as compared to T4, thyroxine-only treatment.

Equally as bizarre and somewhat humorous are the jaw-dropping descriptions patients have reported coming right out of the mouths of their doctors.

- *You will get Mad Cow disease from prescription desiccated thyroid (It's porcine, not bovine).*
- *The T3 in NDT is a narcotic or like speed.*
- *Desiccated thyroid is only given to patients who are "allergic to Synthroid".*
- *If the patient felt better on desiccated thyroid, it had to be due to a preservative in the medication.*
- *It's made from horses.*
- *Just because you feel better on cocaine doesn't mean it's good for you.*
- *It's not made anymore.*
- *Desiccated thyroid is unstable because of the stress of the pigs when they died.*
- *Desiccated thyroid is made from pig testicles.*
- *It's an inferior product made by scooping up the entrails of animals from filthy slaughterhouse floors, and all kinds of bone and germs are in it.*
- *Those who use desiccated thyroid are simply a radical fringe group.*

3. Band-aiding obvious hypothyroid symptoms with more medications or treatments

When patients have complained about ongoing and chronic depression (*a classic hypothyroid symptom*) while on T4-only medications, been put on most any class of prescription antidepressants instead of T3.

Or, like my own mother's tragedy with hypothyroid-caused depression, having electric shock therapy to treat her T4-caused depression, then being put on a tricyclic and becoming apathetic in emotion.

When our cholesterol has risen too high, *(a classic hypothyroid symptom)*, we've been thrust the prescription of our doctor's favorite fermentation-derived or synthetic "statin.".

When our hair started to fall out, or our outer eyebrows almost disappeared *(classic hypothyroid symptoms)*, we've been sent to the nearest Dermatologist who implies it's nothing more than Alopecia Areata.

When we complain of anxiety, emotional swings, an

inability to concentrate, foggy thinking, confusion, etc. *(classic hypothyroid and/or low cortisol symptoms)* we are given our doctors' favorite band-aid psychotropic medication that can contain unneeded fluoride, clash with other medications, make our hypothyroid worse (i.e. lithium), make us fat or can leave classic side effects.

When, like me, we had reactions to activity so bizarre that they incapacitated us *(classic hypothyroid symptom for some of us)*, we have been sent to do unusual, expensive and painful tests, or have been given unfamiliar and far-fetched diagnoses that only served to give meaning to paperwork rather than reality.

When we have complained of ongoing fatigue and poor stamina as compared to others *(classic hypothyroid symptom)*, we've been given the spurious diagnosis of Chronic Fatigue Syndrome or even Fibromyalgia.

When we complain of weight gain that doesn't correspond to our calories consumed, or a severe inability to lose weight *(classic hypothyroid symptoms)*, we are told to simply *eat less, exercise more.* Or like one patient, who was told that she has nothing more than an *'eating problem'*, and *'if she had been in a concentration camp, she wouldn't be fat'.*

4. Failing to understand the reality of adrenal problems, low iron, high RT3

The reality of our adrenals going south accompanying undiagnosed or undertreated hypothyroid has become clearer to patients the past few years, as have treatment strategies.

And no matter how good a doctor becomes in his or her understanding of desiccated thyroid, the correct labs, and dosing by symptoms, failure will continue without understanding the low cortisol factor in such a large body of hypothyroid patients, and how to treat it. Chapters Five and Six detail this common connection.

Also, it's simply all-too-common for us to have non-optimal serum iron, which drives up reverse T3 (RT3). This in turn, makes us more hypothyroid.

Accountability and change

When a dog bites me, I'm going to rightly blame the dog.

Accordingly, when a doctor is patronizing, disrespectful, arrogant, closed-minded, robotic and/or fails to listen to obvious clinical presentation or wisdom straight from the mouth of the patient, *blame lies squarely on the shoulders of the doctor and deserves every ounce of our condemnation and call for change.*

In turn, when a doctor blindly follows the *Big Pharma lie* that a myriad of pills are all that's needed to deal with our ills, it's time to step back. The money-hungry pharmaceutical influence in both medical schools and the doctor's office is both formidable, tragic and lazy. Medical intervention has become focused on pills and ink spots rather than in clinical observation and intuition!

Additional blame can be directed towards the old-boy, big brother influence of a doctor's conservative die-hard medical board or governing body. I still shudder when I think of the transcript I read between a doctor who dared to prescribe desiccated thyroid and dose by symptoms, and his accusing narrow-minded licensing board.

Thyroid patients are calling for serious change in both diagnosis and treatment of hypothyroidism by the medical community. When you make published trials, professional peer pressure, or sales figures the evidence, you are no better than the undressed king who blindly made nakedness the norm. Because we, your patients, are exclaiming The King is Naked! The TSH lab does not correlate to how we feel! Levothyroxine T4-only meds do not fully remove our hypothyroid! Both have resulted in an adrenal problem in too many! What you have been doing is not working, never did, and still doesn't. Stop the Thyroid Madness!

DOCTOR TIDBITS

* Want to stay sick? Patients in nearly every group on the internet have reported that most Endocrinologists have served to do just that when it comes to their rigid reliance on T4-only meds and the TSH lab test, as well as their disdain for your own wisdom.

* What's a Good Doctor? One who respects your own wisdom and intelligence, will do the labs you request, and works with you as a team.

* What's a Bad Doctor? One who talks to you like you couldn't possibly have a brain, refuses to do the labs you request, and thinks only he or she should have a say-so in your health and well-being.

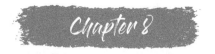

Chapter 8

REASONS YOU MAY BE HYPOTHYROID

Hashimoto's Thyroiditis

Also called "Hashi's" or thyroiditis, this is an autoimmune disorder in which one's immune system attacks its own thyroid cells, causing inflammation and ultimate destruction of your gland over time. It can be one of the most common reasons for your hypothyroid condition. It's two antibodies labs– anti-thyroglobulin and anti-thyroid peroxidase (TPO). Many patients report tightness when they swallow, but some have no symptoms. Patients with Hashi's can vacillate between hypo- and hyper- when the attack grows. There is a genetic predisposition to autoimmune disease, so if you have one, you are more at risk to have others. Check out the book *Hashimoto's: Taming the Beast.*

Other autoimmune thyroid-related causes

In addition to Hashimoto's, there other autoimmune thyroid conditions such as Seronegative Hashimoto's (no antibodies), sub-acute thyroiditis, drug-caused thyroiditis, radiation induced, Riedel's, and Ord's. See these explained in the book *Hashimoto's: Taming the Beast.*

Postpartum, Post-Pregnancy Hypothyroid

Numerous patients report that either Hashimoto's or non-Hashi's hypothyroidism appeared after the birth of a baby, and can also be called "silent thyroiditis" or "post-partum thyroiditis". Some women report they had no indication of an attack or the swings between hypo- and hyper of Hashi's, and simply developed postpartum hypothyroidism. The first signs are easy fatigue, depression (post-partum depression) or reoccurring sicknesses.

Overtreatment for Graves' or Hashi's with Radioactive Iodine

Radioactive iodine (RAI) is commonly used to treat and curb hyperthyroid Graves' disease. It results in the destruction of the thyroid gland. Hypothyroidism appears quickly in some or later in others. Other radiation to the head or neck, including for Hodgkin's disease, can cause hypothyroid.

Bromide Toxicity

Bromide, a chemical compound found in high concentrations in seafood, displaces iodine just like Fluoride, which in turn can cause hypothyroidism. Bromide can be found in commercially prepared breads, some vegetable oils, some citrus sodas, as well as pesticides, some plastics, some dyes, in carpets and mattresses, and more.

Iodine Insufficiency

Since the atoms of thyroid hormones are composed of iodine, there's a strong connection between inadequate iodine intake and hypothyroidism, whether from a lack of iodine in our diet, too much bromide and other toxins, or soil depletion in certain geographical areas.

Selenium Deficiency

Soils can become deficient in selenium, thus food grown in those soils are deficient. And selenium is key for the conversion of the storage hormone T4 to the active hormone T3. Hypothyroidism can result.

Surgery to Remove the Thyroid

When the thyroid gland is surgically removed, called a thyroidectomy, the result will be hypothyroidism. Removal is often the result of hyperthyroidism or thyroid cancer.

Pituitary Gland Failure

When the pituitary gland fails to produce the Thyroid Stimulating Hormone (TSH), hypothyroidism can result, also called Secondary Hypothyroidism. A tumor on the pituitary gland can be one cause, as can a traumatic head injury or disease. Disorders of the hypothalamus, which influences the pituitary, can also cause thyroid hormone deficiency.

Head or Neck Trauma

If any kind of accident caused trauma to the head or neck–even whiplash–secondary hypothyroidism can be the result, as can hypopituitarism.

Cellular Thyroid Hormone Resistance

This rare condition is the result of your bodily tissues and cells being resistant to thyroid hormones and failing to respond. This peripheral resistance could be found in the pituitary gland, or in the outside tissues/cells. High doses of T3-only are required for treatment.

Mutation of the genes DIO1 and/or DIO2

Variations of these genes can result in hypothyroidism by interfering with the conversion of T4 to the active T3.

Pharmaceutical Drug Induced

Lithium, used in the treatment of psychiatric disorders like bipolar, can result in a goiter and/or hypothyroidism by in-hibiting the synthesis of thyroid hormones. Epileptic medications to reduce seizures and the prescription drug Amiodarone used to treat heart arrhythmias, plus Nitroprusside, Perchlorate, and Sulfonylureas can result in hypothyroidism.

Over Consumption of Goitrogens

When eaten in large quantities and consistently, this class of foods can promote goiters and hypothyroidism. They are mostly only a concern when served raw, as cooking may minimize or eliminate goitrogenic potential. Goitrogenic foods include cruciferous vegetables like cauliflower, brussel sprouts and cabbages; dark green leafy vegetables like kale; and root vegetables like turnips, radishes and rutabagas. Soy can especially be a problem if eaten excessively. Eating in moderation is the key rather than eliminating them.

Menopause

Thyroid problems are known to surface at periods of hormonal upheaval and are more common just prior to or during menopause. Statistics state that up to 20% of menopausal women develop hypothyroid problems.

Estrogen dominance

An excess of estrogen in the presence of low progesterone can cause thyroid hormone to be bound and unusable. This can explain why a percentage of peri-menopausal women experience symptoms of hypothyroid for the first time in their lives.

Candida

Yeast Candida is normal in the digestive tract. But there can be an overgrowth from antibiotics, steroids, a high sugar diet, birth control pills, pregnancies, diabetes and more. The immune system then attacks the candida, and the release of chemicals from the attack appears to affect thyroid hormone function.

Aging

Hypothyroidism is one of the most undiagnosed results of aging. In fact, it's not uncommon to watch your elderly loved one become excessively and chronically sleepy, besides depressed and weak. A good discussion with your doctor about thyroid treatment like natural desiccated thyroid, T4/T3 or T3 can be helpful.

Fluoride, Mercury and Environmental Toxins

There is suspicion that the widespread use of fluoride in our water and food may have played a role in the epidemic rise in hypothyroid, since fluoride can interfere with thyroid function. Mercury, especially from our silver fillings, can also play a role in hypothyroidism in susceptible individuals.

Cigarette Smoking

Articles suggest that the toxins in cigarettes interfere with the proper functioning of your thyroid in a multitude of ways, resulting in either hypothyroid or hyperthyroid.

Hepatitis C

The American Journal of Medicine reported in 2004 that if you have chronic Hepatitis C, a blood-borne virus which affects your liver, there is an increased risk of becoming hypothyroid.

Down Syndrome

Along with cardiac disease, it is common to see hypothyroidism in conjunction with Down Syndrome, especially cropping up in childhood.

Autism

Though there is controversy whether autism "causes" or is the "result of" hypothyroidism, an association between the two is common enough to rate mention in this list.

Additional Proposed Causes

- Chronically high cortisol from stress, pushing T4 to convert to Reverse T3 (inactive hormone)
- Family genetic cause of thyroid problems
- Tonsillectomy
- Accumulation of iron in the thyroid gland due to hemochromatosis
- Any problems in the conversion of T4 to T3
- Born without a thyroid: Congenital Hypothyroidism
- Childhood hypothyroid, also called Cretinism
- Asthma and the use of inhaler/expectorants
- Polyunsaturated oils interfere with the release and transport of thyroid
- Excess Cysteine
- Nuclear Plant Exposure

CAUSES OF HYPOTHYROID TIDBITS

* Failing to get enough of certain nutrients like iodine, selenium and zinc can promote a hypothyroid state.

* Daily consumption of soy can cause a goiter and hypothyroidism.

Chapter 9

WHEN YOUR THYROID IS BEING ATTACKED: HASHIMOTO'S DISEASE

B ecoming hypothyroid due to Hashimoto's disease is the most common reason for the condition. Also called Hashi's or chronic thyroiditis, it's a nutty autoimmune attack on your thyroid and the result of your immune system going haywire.

The attack is against your own thyroid tissue rather than bacteria and viruses. It would be akin to turning your sword on your fellow musketeers rather than on the dragons.

The progression of symptoms

How do you know you have it? At first, you may not. The early stages of Hashimoto's Disease can be symptomless. As the attack progresses, the damaged cells of your thyroid become inefficient in converting iodine to thyroid hormones. Thus, your thyroid can compensate by becoming larger, or you can have a sore throat or feel tightness when you swallow. In addition, you might not feel comfortable with that snug collar or turtleneck shirt.

Eventually, you will start to notice the same symptoms of hypothyroid, including poor stamina, easy fatigue, feeling cold, gaining weight, dry hair and skin, constipation, etc. As it progresses, you may feel very hypo- one day, and very hyper- another with a racing heart, palps or anxiety. The hyper is caused by the release of thyroid hormones into your blood due to the destruction. The hypo- is caused by the lessening function of your thyroid due to the destruction.

If your doctor orders lab work, you might see variations in your results, such as being high in the free T3 or free T4 ranges one time, and low the next, or seemingly normal another time, making diagnosing and dosing by labs alone impossible.

The attack and gradual destruction of your thyroid gland can last for years, especially if you are in the hands of a doctor who does fails to do both antibodies tests, or who tells you to *"let it run its course."*

Who has it?

Three out of four individuals with Hashimoto's seem to be women, but men are not immune. Most patients with Hashi's can have a strong family history as well as other autoimmune diseases. Others find themselves with the disease after the birth of a baby, whether they recognize the symptoms or not.

Nancy was surprised to find herself with Hashi's after she had given birth to her first child. She explains:

Over the first 7 months after Eric was born, I was gaining weight rather than losing my pregnancy gain, and I couldn't get past feeling sooo sleepy and blue. My mom told me I had postpartum depression, and time would probably take care of it. So I grabbed a bottle of St. John's Wort to tide me over. A few weeks after that, I was brushing my hair and noticed my neck looked thicker in the front.

Nancy made a quick appointment with her doctor, and she received the diagnosis to explain her symptoms: Hashimoto's Disease.

Lab tests

Since up to 95% of Hashimoto's patients will have antibodies, it can be confirmed by two antibodies labs: **anti-TPO** and **TgAb**. The first antibody, anti-TPO, attacks an enzyme normally found in your thyroid gland, called the Thyroid Peroxidase, which is important in the production of thyroid hormones. The second antibody, TgAb, attacks the key protein in the thyroid gland, the thyroglobulin, which is essential in the production of the T4 and T3 thyroid hormones.

It is unfortunately common for a doctor to only do one test, and you need both, since you can be normal in one test and high in another! The anti-TPO can also be found in hyperthyroidism, aka Graves', as well. So you want to be sure it's Hashi's you have, not simply hyperthyroid. Patients have noticed that saliva does not always accurately detect Hashi's as well as blood tests do.

Occasionally, a doctor will choose non-treatment of your high antibodies, letting it *"run its course"* until it *"stabilizes"*. That's no less like saying *Enjoy feeling like crap for years.*

Additionally, if you let the antibodies run high, which equates to a strong autoimmune attack and inflammation, you can run the risk of both inflammation and autoimmunity spreading to other areas of your body.

Hashimoto's treatment

If the thyroid was attacked long enough before discovery, patients have to treat their hypothyroid the same way that non-autoimmune hypothyroid patients treat--with thyroid medication.

Even on a T4-only treatment (Synthroid, Levothyroxine, etc.), you can have some success in stopping the attack and lowering your antibody levels if you raise high enough. The problem with T4, though, is that it's not adequate and patients usually end up with problems, sooner or later. (Chapter 1)

So what has proven to be a better thyroid treatment? Natural Desiccated Thyroid, or even T4/T3, have proven to do be better for us. And we learned years ago that we have to raise until we are "optimal" on NDT or T4/T3, not just anywhere in the range. Optimal usually always puts the free T3 at the top part of the range and the free T4 midrange. Yet, we also found out that we have to have the right amount of iron and cortisol to get optimal without problems.

Why has the use of thyroid hormones lowered or stopped the antibody attack in patients? I suspect part of it has to do with your immune system. An antibodies attack on your own tissue is, in essence, your immune system going haywire. When you give yourself the thyroid hormones that your body lacks, you then *improve* the health of your immune system, which in turn decreases the production of the crazy antibodies.

Whatever the reason, thyroid patients repeatedly find that holding to too-low doses of thyroid hormones can continue to feed the attack, whereas the more optimal doses finally stop the attack. And with either natural desiccated thyroid or T4/T3, there are far better results both now and throughout one's life

Some randomized placebo-controlled studies suggest that taking Selenium, an essential trace mineral, could help lower the high levels of antibodies, especially the anti-TPO. Recommended doses are 200 - 400 mg daily. But patients have learned that it's meant to be taken in addition to desiccated thyroid or T4/T3, not by itself as a treatment.

Certain patients have noted that their antibodies were present for years even after they had countered the attack with thyroid hormones. This can be a situation where the use of LDN (next heading) is considered.

Pregnancy can be a strong precursor to developing Hashi's, since the increased activity of your immune system can either worsen an autoimmune disease you already have, such as thyroiditis, or cause it to appear. Other researchers suggest that menopause has the same trigger. And patient experiences strongly suggest that hormonal cause of Hashimoto's.

Low Dose Naltrexone (LDN) and Hashimoto's

Naltrexone is an FDA-approved medication that falls under the classification of "Modulators of Opioid and Receptor Activity." In low doses, aka Low Dose Naltrexone, it's been found to be an effective modulator of one's immune system, which is a boon for many Hashi's patients!

As a compounded medication, LDN is usually started at low doses from .5 – 1.5mg, but .5 can be common for Hashimoto's patients. Over many weeks, it's raised slowly until one gets to an amount that produces good results. That can be 3mg, or up to 4.5mg. So it's not about "the higher the better". It's what gives the desired results for you. Typical dosing is twice a day.

In many first-hand reports by Hashimoto's patients, besides medical studies, LDN has either slowed, or halted, the progression of the autoimmune thyroid attack. Hashimoto's patients have reported sleeping better, relief from muscle pain, better digestion, softer skin, lessening of depression, lowering of inflammation, and most importantly...a decrease of antibodies.

The better results from LDN can take longer in some patients than others, so it's important to stick with it, say patients, to get those good results.

Are there side effects from LDN? Many patients report more vivid dreams at night for at least week or longer. Others have reported waking up in the night at first. Overall, patients love what it does for them. If there are too many side effects for a few, they take it only in the morning.

The internet has many good information sites about LDN in the treatment of Hashimoto's.

Removing Gluten from your diet

Just as your antibodies may start attacking your thyroid, they can also attack a substance you consume found in wheat and wheat-similar products: gluten, which unfortunately has cells which can be too similar to thyroid cells.

Gluten can be found in wheat, rye, oats, spelt, barley and others, as well as breads, cereals, pasta, sauces, spices and many processed foods. It's even hidden in my food products you'd least suspect, thus the importance of reading labels.

There will be two ways to have problems with gluten:

1. The autoimmune version of a gluten problem is called **Celiac disease (CD)**. If you eat gluten with Celiac, you end up with a continual attack to your intestinal lining and the tiny villi, resulting in poor absorption of nutrients. This attack can also make Hashimoto's antibodies worse. Testing is usually via the Tissue Transglutaminase Antibodies (tTG-IgA) test, which the majority will have those antibodies. Additionally, your doctor can decide between three other tests.

2. **Non-celiac gluten sensitivity (NCGS)** is a second common reason in Hashimoto's patients in seeing an increase in antibodies. The sensitivity can

cause chronic inflammation, which in turn promotes a worsening of autoimmunity like Hashimoto's, besides the fact that chronic inflammation has serious potential side effects. The diagnosis is based on seeing chronic inflammation via testing of ferritin or C-reactive protein, then testing for Celiac or a wheat allergy with your doctor. If they are negative, there's good reason to believe one has NCGS.

So what's the solution with this unfriendly connection? To completely avoid gluten in your diet.

Iodine and Hashimoto's

Iodine use with Hashimoto's can be a controversial subject among patients. Some report finding themselves with thyroid antibodies which they never had before iodine use. Others report a worsening of current antibodies. *Still others positively report that the use of iodine decreased their antibodies by itself, and if they try to lower their iodine supplementation, their antibodies increase.*

This worsening of antibodies with iodine use can be caused by the detox of bromides, fluorides, and chlorides. Thus, it can be important to not only *go slow and potentially stay* low with iodine, but learn about and use companion nutrients: Vitamin C (3000-10,000 mg), Selenium (200-400 mcg), unrefined Sea Salt (1/2 tsp a day), Magnesium (400 mg - 1200) and B-vitamins with an emphasis on B2 and B3. Companion Nutrients is a term coined by Lynne Farrow, author of the book *The Iodine Crisis: What You Don't Know About Iodine Can Wreck Your Life*

How is Hashitoxicosis related to Hashimotos?

You might call Hashitoxicosis the big mama of the thyroid autoimmune disorders, because you not only have the antibodies anti-TPO and TgAb, but you also have the Graves' Disease antibodies, called TSI, or Thyroid Stimulating Immunoglobulin antibody. The TSI antibody attacks the receptor for the TSH, or thyroid stimulating hormone, then mimics it, causing your thyroid to overproduce thyroid hormones.

A person with this condition has the two opposite spectrums of autoimmune thyroid disease going on: **Hashi's**, which leads to hypothyroid, and **Graves'**, which leads to hyperthyroid. And the swings caused by the multiple antibody attacks can be aggravating. It has been suggested that you dose according to symptoms, i.e. use desiccated thyroid or T3 during the hypo- phase and nothing during the hyper phase. It's difficult, nonetheless.

Another treatment that patients report as successful is with the use of Low Dose Naltrexone mentioned before this.

Accompanying problems

Since Hashi's is an autoimmune disease, patients can be at risk to have other autoimmune diseases, which might include Celiac disease, Pernicious Anemia (vitamin b12 deficiency), or even Addison's, the autoimmune attack of your adrenals. It's individual what will pair with Hashi's. Also, literature states Hashi's can go hand-in-hand with Type 1 Diabetes in susceptible individuals. If you have Hashi's, you can also have food sensitivities and a candida problem.

Bacterial cause of Hashimoto's

Some rare cases of Hashi's may be the result of exposure to particular pathogen (i.e. bad guy) bacteria. The Clinical Microbiology and Infection journal reported in 2001 that there may be a connection between bacteria called Yersinia enterocolitica and certain Hashi's. You can be exposed to these bacteria via tainted meat, unpasteurized milk, untreated contaminated water, or even from the poor hygiene of a food handler. The treatment of choice is with an antibiotic like Doxycycline. Ask your doctor to prescribe a stool lab to discern if you have been exposed to these bacteria.

Bottom line: If your Hashi's is not the result of a bacterial infection, or you don't find success with the antibiotic treatment, patients believe that Hashimoto's can be controlled very successfully if you treat with desiccated thyroid and become optimal (not just "on it"), eliminate gluten and any other offending foods, treat any gut issues, and raise according to the elimination of symptoms, first and foremost.

Want to learn much more about Hashimoto's disease?

Check out the informative book
Hashimoto's: Taming the Beast.

HASHIMOTO'S TIDBITS

* Thyroiditis is a group of disorders that all cause attack and inflammation of the thyroid, and Hashimoto's falls into this group. Some use the term Hashimoto's and Thyroiditis interchangeably.

* Both of two thyroid antibodies need to be tested, not just one, so you can discern if strategies are helping bring both down.

* Vitamin D deficiency will increase your risk of developing Hashimoto's disease, say many research studies.

Chapter 10

JOIN THE YAYA HYPOHOOD PSYCHIATRIST CLUB

Please accept my resignation. I don't want to belong to any club that will accept me as a member.
GROUCHO MARX

Never was a club membership so automatic, vast and dubious as one you might belong to right now along with millions of other women and men worldwide. And how did you acquire this cheeky membership? By being on a T4-only medication like Synthroid, Levoxyl, Eltroxin, Oroxine, levothyroxine, etc, and/or dosed by the TSH lab result, and/or being told by well-meaning but uninformed and robotic doctors that you need...

- To be on antidepressants
- To be on anti-anxiety medications
- To be on lithium (interferes with thyroid function)
- To see a therapist or psychiatrist
- To submit to Electric Shock Therapy, as happened to my own mother

So, because you've always been led to believe that *your doctor knows best*, you've made one of a few choices:

1. Dutifully filled your prescription and popped your anti-depressant, anti-anxiety or other psychotropic pills,
2. Visited your therapist, psychologist or psychiatrist
3. Learned to live with it and coped and coped again. And it's all been in spite of the fact there was a far better medication and treatment which would have prevented the need for most of the psychotropic pills and therapist visits in the first place.

Yet, we were never told.

So along with our physical symptoms of fatigue, poor stamina, dry skin, hair loss, easy weight gain, aches and pains, and/or feeling cold when others were warm...we as a group have had to deal with one or more mental, emotional and psychological symptoms of continuing hypothyroid with unrecognized adrenal problems.

Those symptoms include, but are not limited to:
- Depression
- Anxiety
- Excessive fear
- Bipolar mood swings
- Rage
- Ruminating thoughts
- Chronic irritability
- Paranoia
- Confusion
- Concentration problems
- Memory problems
- Obsessive/compulsive disorders
- Mental aberrations
- Brain fog
- Defensiveness

It's not uncommon for thyroid patients to exclaim that their psychological symptoms can be far more difficult and debilitating than the physical symptoms. Yup, having less stamina than your friends is one thing, but being dependent on yet another medication, or carrying the stigma of an emotional/mental disorder, is another.

Susan, a vibrant chef who chose to stay home when her second child was born later in her life, had been on 0.150 mcg Synthroid for 3 years. She stated:

When I first got on Synthroid, I thought I was going to feel a lot better. My doctor regularly tested my TSH and found what he said was my blue-ribbon dose. Instead, the depression I had before I got on was increasing, and I was so depressed that you couldn't pry me from the house. I didn't enjoy any activities with my husband or my little ones. Holidays were miserable for me, and if I was forced

*to prepare my house for company, it would take me hours
to become motivated enough to do the job. I kept begging
my doctor to see if there was another problem going on,
and all he said was "go see a therapist." I saw two more
doctors, and all I got from them were free samples of
antidepressants and prescriptions for more.*

Mark S., a college student, had symptoms which went
beyond depression. He explained:

*I can't say my life while on 0.125 Levoxyl was horrible,
but I sure wasn't able to keep up with my running buddies
anymore. And something else started to change: I kept
having all sorts of worrisome thoughts in my head. They
would start the minute I woke up and continue until I
went to bed. I couldn't concentrate, couldn't study, and my
thoughts would just roll and roll and roll until I felt like I
was going mad. Felt stupid and alone.*

When hypothyroid patients like Mark and Susan complain
to their doctors about their symptoms,   onto their doctor's
favorite antidepressant,   anti-anxietal,   lithium, or bi-polar
med they go--beginning with the freebies on the shelf from the
friendly and suited pharmaceutical rep. Sound familiar?

Point the finger at a low free T3

Your membership in the club began when your physician
or psychiatrist failed to understand or consider that *mental,
emotional or psychological disorders can be due to inadequate
levels of free T3, the active thyroid hormone.* The low level
can exist *years* before the hypothyroid is detected due to your
doctor's reliance on the faulty TSH lab result. Or it will be
present on T4-only medications where the body is dependent
on the conversion of T4-to-T3 alone, receiving no direct T3 as is
given by desiccated thyroid.

Doctors push you into the club by failing to check thyroid
function with the correct tests, the free T3 and free T4, and
not getting where those two results should fall. *Or, they fail
to recognize the symptoms of adrenal fatigue / HPA dysfunction
or to prescribe the correct diagnostic tests, such as the 24-hour
cortisol saliva test.* It's NOT about blood cortisol testing.

And unfortunately, with their medications come more problems you don't want. Many antidepressants are made up of fluorinated molecules, meaning you are getting the very toxic substance, fluoride, which may be making your thyroid condition worse. Additionally, your medications can clash with other medications, or leave you with other classic side effects, including weight gain.

Depression and hypothyroid

In my contact with hundreds of thousands of thyroid patients over the years, I have repeatedly observed that chronic low-grade depression, and occasionally full-blown depression, is the most common side effect of being on the inadequate thyroxine, T4-only medications. In fact, you can almost guarantee that a large body of patients on thyroxine have been encouraged to be on, or are on, anti-depressant medications. There are some clinical studies which show that long-term use of antidepressants can stress your adrenal function, as well.

Additionally, it doesn't take a rocket scientist to presume that a certain percentage of individuals with depressive disorders who aren't yet on thyroid medications are, in fact, undiagnosed hypothyroid due to the erroneous "normal" range for the TSH lab or the failure to use the correct labs.

My own mother is a classic example of the tragedy of poor assessment or treatment of thyroid function. After she battled clinical depression and anxiety for years while on T4, she relinquished all control of her health to a doctor who gave her Electric Shock Therapy—a treatment which only slightly lessened her chronic depression and dulled her memory and intelligence for the rest of her life. She also remained on the antidepressant Elavil for a lifetime, which made her emotionally flat, along with still being on her Synthroid: the Mutt and Jeff of thyroid treatment.

T3 and your emotional health

Dr. Ridha Arem, in his book *The Thyroid Solution: A Mind Body Program for Beating Depression and Regaining Your Emotional and Physical Health*, states:

Scientists now consider thyroid hormone one of the major "players" in brain chemistry disorders. And as with any brain chemical disorder, until treated correctly, thyroid hormone imbalance has serious effects on the patient's emotions and behavior.

Thyroid hormones thyroxine (T4, as the storage hormone) and triiodothyronine (T3, as the converted, and direct, active hormone) not only play a part in the health of your metabolic, endocrine, nervous and immune system, they in turn have an important role in the health and optimal functioning of your brain, including your cognitive function, mood, ability to concentrate, memory, attention span, and emotions.

On her website, Christiane Northrup, MD wrote about T3 as a neurotransmitter which regulates the action of serotonin and other transmitters against excessive anxiety. She also mentioned that low T3 can be implicated in depression.

Dr. Barry Durrant-Peatfield, in his book *Your Thyroid and How to Keep It Healthy*, explains:

Brain cells have more T3 receptors than any other tissues, which mean that a proper uptake of thyroid hormone is essential for the brain cells to work properly.

Peatfield feels that up to one-half of depression is due to unrecognized hypothyroidism. This figure could be high when you consider the large number of thyroid patients who are suffering from depression while on the inferior treatment of T4-only medications.

One of my favorite articles, *Hypothyroidism Presented as Psychosis: Myxedema* Madness Revisited by Heinrich and Grahm, MD's, outlines the relationship between thyroid disease and psychiatric and psychologic manifestations. They emphatically state:

There is little doubt that thyroid hormone plays a major role in the regulation of mood, cognition and behavior. As a result, persons with thyroid function frequently experience a wide variety of neuropsychiatric sequelae. The range of physical and psychiatric presentations and their potential subtle manifestations make hypothyroidism a diagnosis that is easy to miss. Behavior changes may occur in the absence of classical physical signs and symptoms of the disorder. Pg. 265, Primary Care Companion Journal of Clinical Psychiatry 2003; 5

The additional problem of low cortisol

Just as patients have come to understand the connection between their depression and undertreated hypothyroid, along comes a new wrinkle to be addressed in many: adrenal fatigue/ HPA dysfunction.

Adrenal fatigue means you don't produce enough cortisol, which in turn results in thyroid hormones like T3 "pooling" in the blood—going high with continued hypothyroidism. It is essential that the common combination of hypothyroid and adrenal fatigue be recognized and treated.

Nell had been on Synthroid for eight years, antidepressants for seven, and had many problems. She heard about desiccated thyroid and made the switch. She explained:

I finally made my way up to 2½ grains, held it for five weeks, and found resolution of some my physical symptoms, but I still had others. When I did labs again, my free T3 was over the range, and I felt it was just normal for ME. But just as before, I was still uncomfortable with leaving my house. And my tendency to overreact to things my friends would say to me had not changed. I was calm one moment and raging the next. I also felt like my friends were ganging up on me, and I truly felt one in particular, who has always been an outspoken type of woman, meant to cause me harm. I really thought that! I then heard about low cortisol, did the adrenal self-tests, and it was obvious that they pointed to adrenal fatigue, but I still had to overcome even my fear about THAT.

Nell is an example how low cortisol levels can be an additional culprit, even when you feel you are adequately treated for your thyroid. *Her high free T3 (pooling) along with her psychological symptoms were also suspicious, since low cortisol results in cell receptors failing to adequately receive thyroid hormones from the blood.* The emotional and behavioral symptoms from having low cortisol, which in turn keeps you hypo-, can include the need to avoid leaving one's house, seeking peace and quiet, inability to tolerate stress, low tolerance to loud noises, rage, emotional ups and downs similar to bipolar, panic, obsessive-compulsive tendencies, hypersensitive to the comments of others, phobias, delusions, suicidal ideation, and more.

What's the solution?

Patients and certain informed doctors have learned that if certain mental health symptoms become obvious, it's time to find a doctor who will test your free T3...but you will need to teach most doctors that "optimal", and the removal of all symptoms that doesn't go away, is that which puts the free T3 in the top part of the range...which will lower the TSH below range, and is *not* a problem.

It's also prudent to add the two thyroid antibodies labs, as well as doing the saliva cortisol at four key points during the day. Keep in mind that most doctors will tend to order a urine or blood test, but patients have repeatedly found the 24-hour saliva test to give the best information.

Then watch for optimal cortisol results:

- **Morning wakeup:** *top of the range*
- **Noonish:** *top quarter, towards the bottom part of the quarter*
- **Late afternoon:** *midrange*
- **Bedtime:** *literally bottom of range*

If you find your free T3 mid-range or below, or if you have an autoimmune attack going on against your thyroid (which will make labs useless since you can swing between hypo- and hyper), you need to discuss the addition of Cytomel (synthetic

T3) to your current thyroxine medication.

> *There is a growing body of doctors and researchers who are using T3 as an adjunct to anti-depressive therapy, since improving your T3 levels can raise brain levels of the neurotransmitter's serotonin and norepinephrine to the optimal level they need to be.*

Even better, according to the experience of many, is switching to desiccated thyroid which gives you the entire complement your own thyroid would be giving you–T4, T3, T2, T1 and calcitonin. There are numerous testimonies of patients ridding themselves of chronic depression and other emotional problems when they dosed high enough with desiccated thyroid to put their free T3 towards the top of the range (in the presence of adequate cortisol).

If you find your free T3 at the upper end of the range, or above range, yet mental health issues persist, the missing piece in the puzzle may be the adrenals, pushing FT3 high called pooling. Chapters 5 & 6 provide information patients have learned in the diagnosis and dosing of adrenal insufficiency.

Real life success stories (NDT stands for natural desiccated thyroid)

Joan's story: I was frequently told by my doctors over a ten-year period that I needed to be on antidepressants. I resisted because I didn't want to be like my mother, who'd been on them for years. I finally caved in and tried two brands. One hardly touched my depression. The other worked for three months, then it caused morning depression so bad that I thought I would die. I felt doomed. One particular day, a friend told me about NDT, which her aunt had switched to recently. Since I had been on Levoxyl for more than 10 years, I was curious. I finally found a doctor to put me on NDT, and even as low as 2 grains, I noticed that my depression was disappearing. I am now at 3¾ grains and my depression has totally disappeared.

Nancy's story: Well, I was once on Synthroid for 14 years. My worst times appeared right before my periods, when I would think everyone was ganging up on me. My marriage was in shambles as a result. I also had severe depression during the winter, which I believe is called Seasonal Affective Disorder. I couldn't function during the winter, and my monthly cycles caused me so many problems that I couldn't function most months. Now that I am on NDT, my life has really changed. I can think again. I feel 100% better. I don't dread my periods anymore because my emotions have leveled out. And best of all, I bleed half as much!

Lou's story: For years, I watched my older sis Deb struggle with fatigue. Her doctor finally figured it out and put her on Synthroid. Deb seemed to do better, but she still had depression, and her hair kept getting thinner and thinner. Then it was my turn! I became hypothyroid about four years after my sister. But I did some research on the internet, found out about desiccated thyroid, and got on NDT. Once I got over 3 grains, I felt SO much better and could run circles around my sister. Luckily, she is looking into getting off her Synthroid and onto desiccated thyroid like me.

Judy's story: This is embarrassing, but I've always been very obsessive-compulsive. There have always been certain ways I have to do things around the house, and I'm anxietal if my husband does it differently. When it thunders really loud, I feel better by reciting the alphabet over and over. I've been on Levothyroid for 16 years, since I was 18. I have never had the energy of my friends. I heard about Janie and a group she has, and found a doctor to put me on NDT. He refused to let me go higher than 2 grains, so I found another doctor 1½ hours away from my house. She let me go higher. And to my shock, I am not anywhere NEAR as OCD as I've always been. I am thinking that all along, it was a thyroid symptom that the Levothroid never took away! I am so excited.

Michelle's story: I think I have been to more than nine doctors in the past few years, and every one of them told me I needed to be on antidepressants. It only made me cry even more, as I read so many bad stories about them. I am now on NDT, and no longer feel depressed or anxietal.

Lucille's story: I was depressed for eleven years before discovering that I had a thyroid problem–just like my mother. I had been on a variety of antidepressants for at least six of those eleven years. When I was on Levoxyl and later Synthroid when I moved and changed doctors, my depression got even worse. Because my husband kept liquor in the house, I started drinking. I'm now on 4½ grains desiccated thyroid, and my depression has lifted! Who would have guessed? Yes, I stopped drinking and feel better than I have in a decade.

Mrs. R's story: I have always had problems with what they call suicide ideation. I wasn't actively suicidal, but I sure have been passively suicidal, thinking about it and being careless. I've been on antidepressants off and on, too, including Elavil, which turned me into a zombie. I finally got my doc to do some blood work. He said I was hypothyroid–put me on Levothyroxine. It did NOTHING for me. NOTHING. I then joined an internet thyroid support group, heard about desiccated thyroid and switched. I am actually feeling better than ever! I'm excited what more will happen to me as I raise my free T3 levels.

Steve's story: I am a student in college. Ever since I was about 13, I've had episodes of mania and depression. I could barely get along with my mother, and I spent many days living with a strict aunt and uncle. I thought weight lifting would make a difference, but it didn't. My doctor put me on Synthroid when I was a senior in high school. It didn't help at all. And when I went away to college, I had trouble keeping friends due to my mood swings, besides being dog-tired and I ached. The university doctor had me raise my thyroid medication.

It did nothing. I heard about NDT and started it. I had a terrible reaction to it, and through getting on the internet, found out about adrenal fatigue. I am currently on Cortef, started my NDT again, and am actually feeling like an even-keeled human being again. Thank you.

Pam C's story: I have had depression for 18 years and even had to spend time in a mental hospital in Dallas. I was on Levoxyl, too. Three times during that time, when I questioned if my thyroid problem might be causing all this, all I got was "no" because my TSH was normal and I needed to see a psychiatrist and stick with my antidepressants. When I got a computer for Christmas, I started doing research using Google and found out that a low T3 causes depression, and that NDT might stop it since it has direct T3. I was dancing, let me tell you. I promise that the first day I took it, I started to feel better. I wish I had known about this years ago. Not one doctor told me anything. Not one.

Cindy's story: I can only speak for me, but since I started on NDT three months ago, I still get depressed at times. But now, I seem to be able to pull myself out of it! The depression is also much lighter. I am looking forward to more progress.

G.R's story: I was diagnosed with hypothyroid 8 years ago and put on Synthroid. Six years ago, I was diagnosed with Body Dysmorphic Disorder and I've been on several psychotropic medications that did not help. It was my mom who told me what she had heard about NDT, so I found a doctor who would let me get on it, then switched to a DO who would let me get higher. I am now on 5 grains, plus 27½ mg Cortef (hydrocortisone). I am shocked to report that I no longer have depression or anxiety attacks, and I don't feel hideous anymore. It's a miracle really.

Listening to the success stories

Those stories above only barely touch the surface of success by those who moved from T4-only medications and dosing by the TSH... to a T3 treatment or desiccated thyroid.

They also dosed **not** by the TSH, but by the elimination of symptoms with a Free T3 and Free T4 as guides. Optimal has always put the free T3 towards the top and free T4 midrange. Both. But you have to have good iron and cortisol to get there without problems.

So don't despair if you are a bonafide and oh-so-privileged member of the Yaya Hypohood Psychiatrist Club. You can switch your membership to an inactive status by getting on desiccated thyroid, or at the very least, adding T3 to your T4-only medication...and achieving optimal.

YAYA HYPOHOOD TIDBITS

Turns out that a certain percentage of patients with the anxiety disorder called Agoraphobia (fear of leaving the house or being in public) also have a thyroid problem.

* Hashimoto's can be common in those with schizophrenia. [18]

* Some cases of Bipolar may have a strong connection to hypothyridism[19], as well adrenal fatigue / low cortisol.

* Paranoia and overeactiveness is a common problem with adrenal fatigue members in social media groups.

---

18 https://www.ncbi.nlm.nih.gov/pmc/articles/PMC3978977/
19 https://www.ncbi.nlm.nih.gov/pubmed/21808723/

Chapter 11

THE 10 BIGGIES: THE MOST COMMON MISTAKES

Bloopers, blunders and miscalculations: all common when treading a new path. Patients who've walked the better path with thyroid or adrenal treatment have experienced all of them. My own learning curve was having a doctor start me on ¾ grain of natural desiccated thyroid. Not a huge mistake, since it can be wise to have a low introductory dose to help your body adjust to the direct T3, a very powerful thyroid hormone.

But what she did next was the biggie: *she left me on that ¾ grain for nine weeks before I saw her again.* A huge mistake! Due to the feedback loop, my pituitary gland thought my thyroid was now producing a bit more hormones, and via the TSH, it told my actual poorly-producing thyroid to produce even less. Thus, my hypothyroid symptoms came back with a *vengeance.* The first evidence was a menstrual period that lasted twice as long as usual.

1. Staying on a starting dose too long: Just like my example above, it's common for doctors to put you on a safe low starting dose, but leave you on it far too long, i.e. until the next six-week or eight-week follow-up.

The result? Your body thinks your thyroid has suddenly produced more hormones. And via the TSH from your pituitary gland, your thyroid is told to decrease its already-lowered production. So you become even more hypothyroid than you started.

We have learned that though one grain is a beneficial and safe amount to start with for most, especially in the presence of adequate cortisol, it's not a good amount to remain on much longer than two weeks or less without raising by at least one-half grain. Patients continue with ½ grain raises every two weeks. Some may find an optimal amount in the 2+ grain area, but most others will need more, and to slow down as they approach two to three grains to give the T4 in desiccated thyroid a full four to six weeks to fully build, then to test.

If you have to start as low as 30 mg, either due to your doctor's lead or because of adrenal issues, it's even more crucial to begin raising by the end of the first week. With adrenal dysfunction being treated with cortisol, the raises may need to be in smaller amounts, even if close together.

2. Not raising until one is optimal: This is a common occurrence which can happen anywhere along the way of your desiccated thyroid dosing. Patients will be on inadequately low doses due to:

a. *Being held on a starting dose too long.*
b. *Being bound by the directives of a TSH-obsessed doctor*
c. *Failing to get a raise of desiccated thyroid until the "next lab work", which can be too far away.*
d. *Following an inaccurate Synthroid-to-desiccated thyroid conversion equivalence chart, which leaves you under-dosed.*
e. *Being forced to lower a dose due to a high free T3 with continuing hypo- symptoms, which is "pooling"- a sign of low cortisol and needs treatment. (Chapter 5 and 6.)*
f. *Being afraid to go higher.*

For example, a patient makes her way up to one, or one-and-a-half grains (60 - 90mg) and notices good improvements and feels better... yet fails to raise to be OPTIMAL. What is optimal? We see it when the free T3 is at the top part of the range, and the free t4 is midrange. Both.

What happens if we don't get optimal? It all backfires,

sooner or later, with a return of hypothyroid symptoms. The individuality is when those symptoms will return.

It's estimated that the daily average secretion of thyroid hormones in individuals without thyroid disease is 94 – 100 µg T4 and 10 - 22 µg T3[20]. Since US-made desiccated thyroid has 38 mcg of T4 and 9 mcg of T3 per one grain (60 or 65 mg), the above amounts equate to about three to five grains of desiccated thyroid. And sure enough, a certain body of hypothyroid patients have noticed that their optimal dose ends up in the three to five grain range before ridding themselves of symptoms.

Or, some may find themselves optimal in the 2+ grain area. Or some higher than 5 grains. It's very individual. Bottom line, though, it's always about being optimal!

It can also be very wise to check cortisol levels, since low cortisol can prevent thyroid hormones from making it to the cells, thus pooling in the blood. With low cortisol, you will still have symptoms even in the three-to-five grain dosage range, or even be unable to reach that area due to hyper-like symptoms.

3. Thinking hyper symptoms are only from taking too much: Granted, a patient can take too much desiccated thyroid and become hyper, revealed by a higher heart rate or blood pressure, sweating, anxiety, shakiness, etc. But if you have hyper- like symptoms on doses less than three grains, there's a good chance the cause is from either *struggling adrenals and/or low iron*. Both of these situations cause problems which the NDT or T3 will reveal. So it can be wise to get your cortisol levels checked via a 24- hour cortisol saliva test (*http://www.tinyurl/saliva-cortisol*), iron with all four iron labs (Chapter 13), and your RT3, which low iron kicks up. (Chapter 13)

4. Failing to multi-dose: It's a common feature of many popular medications to take a pill once a day. Those on any T4-only medication, which is a storage hormone with a long lifespan, do just that. Some thyroid patients who take desiccated thyroid also take it once a day, in the morning.

---

[20] www.thyroidmanager.org/

But over time, it's possible the once-a-day strategy may backfire, leaving you with afternoon fatigue and/or stressed adrenals. Plus it's not what a healthy thyroid would be doing—dumping all its hormone at one time. The direct T3 is immediate, peaking about two hours after you take it, and then beginning its fall with a shorter life-span that T4. So dividing your dose makes sense.

For example, a person on three and one-half grains might take two grains in the morning, and 1 ½ by early to mid-afternoon. Occasionally, some might have reason to take it three times a day, but it's less common.

Another benefit of multi-dosing is that it's far less stressful on your adrenals, which is especially crucial if you have sluggish adrenal function and still trying to find your optimal dose of cortisol supplementation.

5. Swallowing thyroid with estrogen, calcium or iron: Unfortunately, when you swallow your desiccated thyroid at the same time you swallow foods or supplements which contain calcium, iron, excess fiber, or even estrogen, a certain amount of the direct T3 in your thyroid pill will be become bound and unusable in the mix. Not all. Some.

How far apart should they be taken? Opinions vary. Perhaps 2 hours minimum. It is acceptable to have food in your stomach, though, when you take your desiccated thyroid, as long as they don't contain the above.

When avoiding calcium supplements, you have to watch out for calcium-fortified orange juice, as well as taking calcium carbonate over-the-counter products like Tums or Rolaids.

> *We used to think that doing NDT or T3 sublingually under the tongue would be ideal, thinking it wouldn't get to the stomach. But I lean to believe that's wrong, and that we do swallow "some" of it.*

6. Thinking desiccated thyroid is not working when an issue arises: The brilliance of desiccated thyroid is that it contains direct T3, also called *triiodothyronine*. It's the most powerful of the thyroid hormones. Because of that power, it can initially aggravate certain conditions as they are exposed to the T3.

An example is my benign heart condition called Mitral Valve Prolapse. I noted that with each raise, I would have consistent palpitations from the mitral valve. But within five days, my heart would calm down and come out stronger.

Another patient got itchy when she got on desiccated thyroid, and was so determined to blame it that she got off, got back on Synthroid...and is still itchy. We have since learned from a few patients that the itchiness went away as they continued to raise their desiccated thyroid until they were optimal.

7. Adding T4 to desiccated thyroid: The vast majority of patients (who have good iron and cortisol) report they achieve excellent health, stamina and energy on desiccated thyroid alone, especially when they have taken the time to raise and find their optimal dose. Optimal seems to put the free T3 at the top area and free T4 midrange Both. Adding T4 is rarely needed.

Others may be adding T3 to their lower dose of NDT due to having high RT3, and working on the causes. That can work.

8. Going up with dosages too fast: I remember vividly the following experience on an internet thyroid patient group: a male patient was prescribed desiccated thyroid, and on his own, he raised it one grain per week, reaching six grains by the sixth week. Ouch. He started to find himself heavily overdosed with symptoms to match, including high anxiety and shakiness. He had to cease taking any thyroid for a few weeks to allow the T4 to fall. His doctor then restarted his dosage at one grain, and a more prudent dose raise began.

Namely, patients have learned that after being on a starting dose for about two weeks (one grain, for example), they can start raising their dosage by ½ grain or so every two weeks. They also note that when they 'near" three grains (are somewhere in the 2-grain area), it's time to hold each dose several weeks to see its T4-to-T3 conversion results.

9. Not understanding that "feeling good" on NDT or T4/T3 doesn't mean we are "optimal": We have noticed that most of us will feel good on lower, non-optimal doses of NDT or T4/T3...for awhile. Then some will stop there, thinking *"I'm at the right dose"*. But not necessarily!! Stopping before optimal can mean our bodies will use up the T4/T3 too quickly. Thus, we are destined to see it backfire with a return of hypothyroid symptoms.

The amount that doesn't backfire is what we call an "optimal" amount—that which puts the free T3 towards the top area of the range, and the free T4 midrange.

10. Not understanding the problem of excess Reverse T3 (RT3): A growing body of patients who have either high cortisol, low iron, or inflammation, can see T4 convert to excess RT3. Then their Free T3 levels drop since RT3 will hog the cell receptors, preventing T3 from getting in

And the challenge then becomes finding a doctor who understands that RT3 needs to be tested and treated. Where should RT3 be in any range? The bottom two numbers (or lower), and only occasionally the 3rd number above the bottom, is where we consistently see RT3 in those who don't have an RT3 problem. Because of these observations, we stopped doing the ratio between the Free T3 and RT3 to discern an RT3 problem.

TEN BIGGIES TIDBITS

* Since hypothyroidism can result in "brain fog" and mistakes in treatment are a result, find a trusted friend or loved one to help you go through this book. Also consider taking this book to the appointment with bookmarks.

* Thinking your doctor knows more than you do, and failing to demand respect for your own subjective experience and wisdom in the doctor's office, can keep you sick.

Chapter 12

T3 IS THE STAR OF THE SHOW

*The man who follows the crowd will usually get no further
than the crowd. The man who walks alone is
likely to find himself in places no one has been.*
ALAN ASHLEY-PITT

Most legendary bands have a lead singer who draws the most attention of their fans. And when it comes to the ensemble of thyroid hormones, the one with the lead gold star on its door by thyroid patients is T3, aka triiodothyronine (try-i-oh-doh- thy-ro-neen).

T3, an iodine-based hormone, is part of a family of five well- known performing hormones produced by a healthy thyroid: T4, T3, T2, T1 and calcitonin. Together, they all work as smoothly and harmoniously as a well-tuned chorus for the optimal performance of your body. In the human body, some literature states the storage hormone T4 is approximately 93% of the total thyroid production, with T3 coming in at 7% and smaller amounts of T2, T1 and calcitonin. Others will state it's an 80/20% split for T4/T3.

T3 deserves the academy award

T3 is the most biologically active, life-giving hormone made by your thyroid, being around four to eight times more powerful than the storage hormone T4. It makes its appearance in your body two ways: first, from the conversion of T4 to T3 by the removal of an iodine atom, and second, by being made endogenously, meaning directly.

T3 positively affects every cell, tissue, and organ in your body. It plays a critical role in your energy levels, stamina, immune strength, hair and skin health, brain function, metabolism, liver function and body temperature. T3 has a special role in the health of your heart as well as your emotional and mental well-being.

The presence of direct T3 (as compared to conversion from T4), *is exactly why a large and growing body of patients are finding natural desiccated thyroid gives them far more benefit than being on a T4-only.* At the very least, even being on a synthetic T4/T3 combination is far sweeter than T4 alone.

T3 and the health of your heart

Studies frequently reveal the strong connection between the thyroid hormone T3 and its influence on a healthy heart rate, good blood pressure and vascular resistance–the latter which refers to your body's ability to push blood through your circulatory system. T3 plays a strong role in normalizing cholesterol levels. Conversely, low levels of T3 can coincide with a poorly functioning heart rate, rising blood pressure, and atherosclerosis--the hardening of your arteries

This strong connection between the T3 thyroid hormone and your cardiovascular health has not gone unseen by thyroid patients over the years, even if they didn't understand what they were seeing.

At first, Cathy was stymied by what happened to her 68-year-old mother when she had heart surgery, but came to an important conclusion ten years later. She explained:

On my mother's side of the family, I never heard any stories about heart problems. My grandparents died from old age. And my mom's weight gain wasn't unusual to me since my grandmom had been a little overweight as the owner of a bakery. Yet when my mother was in her late 60's, and had been on Synthroid about 35 years, she had to have a balloon angioplasty. I was told it was done to open up a narrowed artery from her rising cholesterol. And it seemed really odd to me. But I figured it out a decade later when I

*joined a thyroid group. A lot of other thyroid patients were
talking about their own high cholesterol when on those
T4 pills. And others mentioned heart problems. One girl
said she was in heart failure in her 40's while being on
Synthroid, and it was totally different now that she was on
desiccated thyroid! It was like a light bulb went off in my
head about my mom.*

A familiar pattern is true for a large body of hypothyroid
patients who are on T4-only medications as they age: unfailing
weight gain, rising cholesterol and heart issues. Even in 1976,
when Dr. Broda Barnes wrote *Solved: The Riddle Heart Attacks*,
he clearly saw a strong connection between hypothyroid and
heart disease.

**And since patients have found their hypothyroid to continue
while on T4-only medications, rising cholesterol is the norm as
can be towards cardiovascular disease as we age.**

Conversely, those who switch to desiccated thyroid with
its direct T3, and who raise not by the TSH lab result but
according to the free T3 and free T4, report a firm lowering
of their cholesterol levels and much improved cardiovascular
health. Sharon tells her inspiring story:

*I had been on Levothyroxine for 16 years when I heard
about Desiccated thyroid from a thyroid support group
on the internet. I was so impressed that when I went back
to our family doctor to talk about my labs, I was going to
insist on switching. He's an older doctor and knew about
natural thyroid. Lucky me, because he was very friendly
about me being on it. This was also the appointment
where I found out that my cholesterol was 305! I picked
up my pills that afternoon, and started the Stop the
Thyroid Madness book the next day. I told him how I
wanted to raise it based on what I had learned from other
people in my shoes, and he gave me enough until the next
appointment, and asked me to report in every three weeks.
When I tested my cholesterol again several months later,
it was down to 198!! I did nothing different other than
switching to natural thyroid!*

Sharon's story is similar to thousands of thyroid patients who make a switch to a desiccated thyroid product. And a visit to one of numerous internet thyroid patient groups attest to cardiovascular improvement in a large body of thyroid patients. To see a plethora of articles on the connection between T3 and heart health, just use your favorite search engine and type in *triiodothyronine cardiovascular*.

T3's role against depression

Feeling chronically sad? Have problems feeling excited about your life? Studies show a strong relationship between your free T3 level ("free" referring to the available and unbound of the total T3) and the occurrence of depression and feelings of emotional numbness; namely, *the lower your free T3 levels, the higher the incidence of depression and related emotions of apathy.*

As outlined in Chapter 10, chronic depression is quite common for those on T4-only medications where the only T3 patients get is from conversion. But when patients switch to a desiccated thyroid treatment with its direct T3, Or add T3 to their T4 and find their "optimal", you hear a multitude of subjective reports about the improvement and/or removal of the chronic depression. Patients then report a successful end to antidepressants.

Biologically, thyroid hormones, especially the active and life-giving T3, interact with brain receptors and make the brain more sensitive in favor of norepinephrine or serotonin. Norepinephrine, a neurotransmitter, plays a role in your alertness, memory and the balancing of your mood. Serotonin regulates mood and emotion.

According to numerous studies which report on the use of T3 in combating depression, the improvement occurred whether the patient was considered hypothyroid or not. One is left to question whether the diagnosis against hypothyroid was accurately made. The occurrence of undiagnosed hypothyroid is widespread, perpetual and odious due to the obsessive reliance on the faulty TSH. So in reality, there might be a vast percentage of depressed patients who are quite hypothyroid.

With T3 added to your anti-depressant, it's proposed that the T3 accelerates the effects of the anti-depressant. Even more concisely, it may be treating the very reason for the depression in the first place–a low free T3 due to hypothyroid. **There are simply numerous examples of patients whose depression completely resolved when their hypothyroid was correctly diagnosed and optimally treated with desiccated thyroid, or at the least, a synthetic T4/T3 combination or T3 alone.**

Bottom line, the addition of T3 in the treatment of depression has a good track record of being safe, practical, and inexpensive, whether taken alone or combined with T4 as in desiccated thyroid, or simply as an adjunct to antidepressants. And it works.

In the Oct. 2000 issue of *The Annal of Pharmacotherapy* 34 (10):1142-45, the following abstract is a good example of what occurs with many hypothyroid and depressed patients when they have a thyroid treatment that includes direct T3 (and underscores why forcing the body to live for conversion alone with T4-only can be a disaster):

OBJECTIVE: To describe a patient with longstanding depression and hypothyroidism who had marked mood improvement only after triiodothyronine (T3) was added to her thyroxine (T4) replacement therapy.

CASE SUMMARY: A 50-year-old white woman had a long history of depression and documented hypothyroidism since 1991. Despite treatment with T4 with dosages up to 0.3 mg/d, she continued to be depressed, have symptoms of hypothyroidism, and have a persistently elevated thyroid-stimulating hormone concentration. Addition of a low dose of T3 to her regimen resulted in significant mood improvement.

DISCUSSION: The relationship between hypothyroidism and depression is well known. It is possible that this patient's long history of depression may have been a consequence of inadequately treated hypothyroidism, due either to poor patient compliance or resistance to T4. Nevertheless, her depression responded to addition of a low dose of T3 to her regimen. This case emphasizes the importance of screening depressed patients for hypothyroidism. Her clinical course also suggests that depression related to hypothyroidism may be more responsive to a regimen that includes T3 rather than to replacement with T4 alone. This is consistent with the observation that T3 is superior to T4 as adjuvant therapy in the treatment of unipolar depression.

CONCLUSION: Depressed patients should be screened for hypothyroidism. In hypothyroid patients, depression may be more responsive to a replacement regimen that includes T3 rather than T4 alone. Therefore, inclusion of T3 in the treatment regimen may be warranted after adequate trial with T4 alone.

Alongside the numerous study results showing the efficacy of T3 treatment in depression, there are also several references to the successful use of T3 in the treatment of anxiety, Body Dysmorphic Disorder, Bipolar, Obsessive-Compulsive, Suicide Ideation, to name a few. This is huge!

Two scenarios which might require T3-only treatment (or mostly T3)

No matter how beneficial patients have found desiccated thyroid to be in the complete reversal of hypothyroid symptoms, there can be **two problems** that a certain percentage of patients experience:

1) Thyroid Hormone Resistance (THRB gene)

Imagine that your vehicle's gas tank has plenty of fuel, but your car is unable to make use of it. That is akin to *"thyroid hormone resistance,"* usually due to a mutation of the THRB gene. Luckily, it's rare, but I have noticed that there seem to be more of it coming from those in or from western Europe.

Having thyroid hormone resistance means the tissues in your body are resistant to the effects of thyroid hormone. May look great or even high, but the TSH is not low, as it would be with high levels of T4.

As a result, people with this active mutation end up needing supraphysiologic high levels of desiccated thyroid and added T3, or just T3 since T4 may be at toxic high levels, and only dose based on the resolution of symptoms.

2) High Reverse T3 (RT3)

In most humans, and in any situation where one's body needs to conserve energy such as illness, surgery or an accident, the thyroid will properly convert any excess T4 to the inactive Reverse T3 in order to lower one's metabolism and to concentrate on the problem at hand. Even having the flu can cause this conversion.

But sometimes for us as thyroid patients, one's body makes far too much RT3 for other reasons:

1) inadequate levels of iron   *see labs online*
2) high levels of cortisol
3) chronic inflammation or infection

Or, if we are detoxing high heavy metals, dealing with Lyme disease, exposed to mold, up goes the RT3. Even beta blockers can, in higher doses, cause high RT3[21]. On and on.

Picture running water down a street heading towards a side drain, but the water is also picking up a mess of twigs and branches along the way, until the drain becomes so clogged with twigs and branches that water can no more fall down the drain. This is akin to what happens when your body is making excessive RT3–it lowers the amount of T3 that can get into and interact with your cells.

How to discern high RT3 before you test it

1. The first clue comes with the subjective experience of feeling toxic or more hypothyroid as you try to raise your thyroid medications. Or, as patients report firsthand: not quite feeling right, strange reactions, not getting benefits like others do, a low temperature, anxiety, etc.
2. Another clue comes with your most current lab results.

---

[21] https://www.ncbi.nlm.nih.gov/pubmed/1688102

If you find yourself with a high-in-the-range Free T4 and a low-range free T3, it strongly implies that conversion is heading the direction of excess RT3, which lowers Free T3. Only much later will T4 fall due to its excess conversion to RT3.

How patients improve their high RT3

1. The first answer is obvious: **treat the causes** which I listed previous to this.
2. **Support your liver.** Since the bulk of RT3 is made in the liver, some have lowered their high RT3 by using a good liver support, especially those made from **Milk Thistle seeds.** Dandelion Root and Yellow Dock are also good liver supports. With Milk Thistle, you may have to double or triple the recommended bottle amount to get the lowered RT3. *But note: Milk Thistle can lower your iron levels a bit, too, so patients are adding iron to their supplementation*
3. **Test your selenium:** there is a lot of research which proves that low selenium can increase RT3. If low, 200-400 mcg is said to be safe.
4. **Going on T3-only:** T3-only dosing can have its challenges, since there's no T4 to convert to T3 for you. But since it's converting to excess RT3 anyway, it can be necessary to use T3 and multi-dose.

Switching to and dosing with T3-only

If you choose to use T3-only for thyroid treatment (and your doctor agrees with it, which is sometimes challenging), we found it can be wise to start on low amounts, raise in small amounts, and multi-dose it while working on improving other issues. Work with your doctor on this, please.

Generally, starting on T3 can be like this:

1. If someone is very sensitive or has a lot of issues, they start low, such as 2.5, 2.5, and 2.5mcg every four hours starting first thing in the morning.

2. If someone isn't quite as sick, but wants to be on more T3, they might do 5, 5, and 5 mcg, split into three doses, four hours apart. Some even start on 20 or 25 mcg total without a problem, split to three doses every four hours apart.
3. Some people are adding T3 to their lowered NDT. So two doses are T3, and the third is the NDT.

Like the mitral value prolapse I have, which makes one's heart sensitive, starting on these lower doses gives the heart time to adjust, if needed. The multi-dosing times can be figured out by paying attention to symptoms. Some notice the T3 wearing off sooner than four hours, so move to three hours. Others do fine on a four-hour spread.

Some patients add an extra dose of T3
(such as 2.5mcg) to bedtime, assisting detoxing,
cellular repair, and better sleep.

Nothing about dosing T3 is an exact science. It can be an individual trial and error process.

Bottom line, we're trying to replace with T3 at the same time T4 is falling (if we were once on T4-only, NDT or T4/T3 treatments. Additionally, if our RT3 was high, our cells receptors might still be overrun with RT3 and thus, we won't be receiving all the T3. So we can feel more hypo- at times, or temps may go a bit weird after a raise. It eventually evens out.

Every five days to a week, after establishing the multi-dosing routine mentioned previous and needing more T3, patients continue to add T3 to first the morning dose, then the next, keeping the morning slightly higher than noon, and the 3rd dose a little lower. But this is only if a raise doesn't cause a racing heart or palps. That could be a sign we weren't ready for a raise.

T3 has a short half-life, thus the ability to raise every five or so days.

What amount of T3 is enough

Generally, we've noticed in each other for years that optimal on T3-only puts the free T3 right towards the top area of the range, and in some, slightly over...and neither with hyper-like symptoms. Or, if there is a mix of T3 with a lowered amount of NDT (or T4), it's still towards the top area of the range as long as there is no bad reaction, palps, or high heartrate.

Again, *one has to have the right amount of cortisol* to achieve a true optimal result with the free T3 without bad results. If cortisol is low when starting on T3, or someone isn't yet on the right amount of cortisol supplementation, patients can't raise enough, because the free T3 will pool, looking right but not actually getting to the cells. So they stay lower, and work on getting the right amount of cortisol.

The amount of T3 medication which results in optimal (in the presence of the right amount of cortisol) will vary from individual to individual! In some, in can happen around 50 mcg, but in others, as high as the lower 100's...and all in between. That variance in amounts of T3 meds is why we have to frequently test the free T3. Other clues can be obtained by watching your temperature and pulse, i.e. if they go too high, it may be too much.

Clearing of high RT3 with T3-only

If someone feels they want to clear a high RT3 with T3-only, it seems to take a minimum of eight weeks to fully get a high level down. Yes, it goes down, but those weeks are needed in some to get it all the way down.

Some patients theorize that they may need higher amounts of T3 in order to bombard the cell receptors and to clear out the excess RT3. This will then become too much, and patients report a temporary and sudden high heartrate/blood pressure and adrenaline surges. T3 is then reduced quite rapidly. But mentioning this is not a recommendation

Optimal dosing seems to put the free T3 is at the top of the range or slightly over (in the presence of adequate cortisol supplementation). Having a higher range FT3 can be necessary while on T3-only to compensate for the inability to receive T3 from the conversion of T4, report patients.

It's also been noted that when patients are optimal on T3, their adrenals seem to begin healing. How was that discovered? By suddenly noting high cortisol symptoms on the amount of HC they once needed after doing their DATS.

Free T4 and TSH on T3

Once on T3 long enough and optimally, you will see a low TSH and a low Free T4. The lowered T4 means less RT3, as well. Sometimes doctors are concerned with the low FT4, but we've never found it to be a problem.

Brands and kinds of T3

All T3 products are synthetic T3-only, and there are a variety of brand names and locations they are made. Cytomel is often a favorite of many doctors in the US, as well as by patients. But some generics work just as well and are cheaper! I have personally done well with a generic brand. See the Resources at the end of this book.

Compounded T3 is available by prescription, but it's usually slow release, and that isn't always ideal. Even *Dr. John C. Lowe felt that time-released T3 is not a wise choice, since calcium in the intestines can bind the T3 which is hanging around longer due to being 'time-released'.*

How long patients stay on T3-only

The length of time patients stay on T3 is an individual call, based on how long it takes to lower RT3, or whether there are ongoing issues which will push RT3 back up if one got off T3, such as chronic inflammation, infections, or chronic high stress which will cause high cortisol.

If a time comes that we feel we have adequately treated the causes of high RT3, patients may be ready to consider a slow tapering of the T3 while adding back in desiccated thyroid or T4 to the T3. Since one grain of desiccated thyroid (with both direct T3 and conversion of T4 to T3) is roughly equivalent to 25 mcg T3, the latter can slowly be dropped as one grain is replaced. The "slow" drop of T3 is to give T4 time to convert.

A few patients stay on T3 for life if there are issues they can't resolve.

> *Did you know that even some cardiologists report
> using T3 to help their heart patients?
> Same with psychiatrists who report using T3
> for their patients' depression. Hopefully you can work
> with your doctor about this!*

The half-life of T3

Half–life refers to the amount of time it takes for half the T3 in your body to fall in such a way that you might feel it. And thyroid patients have discovered that the half-life of T3 depends on how hypothyroid you are, i.e. the more hypo- you are, the shorter the T3 lasts, which is why most have to dose no more than 4 hours apart when first on T3 or desiccated thyroid.

Conversely, the more adequately treated you are, the longer the T3 lasts, which subjectively can seem like many more hours after your last dose! The author of this book, who has been adequately treated on desiccated thyroid, notices that even when she forgets her morning dose, she'll feel fine until mid-afternoon. At that point, she may notice sleepiness, and then realizes *"Oops. I forgot to take my morning dose and my T3 is now low enough to feel it!"*

Becoming educated about the role of T3 in our thyroid treatment has been a major boon in our road to better health and energy. Or as my uncle would quote, "it's the greatest thing since sliced bread".

T3 TIDBITS

* The attack on one's thyroid due to having Hashimoto's antibodies can push RT3 up due to the inflammation.

* T3 raises your Sex Hormone Binding Globulin (SHBG), and men may need to look into testosterone supplementation as a result.

* T3 supplementation can cause estrogen levels to drop a bit.

* 25 mcg of T3 is roughly equivalent to one grain of desiccated thyroid.

* T3 might help prevent liver cancer, says this research. http://cancerres.aacrjournals.org/cgi/content/abstract/60/3/603

* FT3 peaks in "approximately" 2 hours with desiccated thyroid, and in "approximately" 4 hours on straight T3.

Chapter 13

IMPORTANT ODDS AND ENDS RELATED To BEING HYPOTHYROID

L ike a cat walking gracefully along the edge of a fence, healthy bodies are always in a state of balance. The fit action of one organ can affect the stable reactions of another in a perfect equilibrium.

On the other side of the coin, when one organ becomes diseased or there are bodily deficiencies, imbalance occurs. And in hypothyroid patients, whether from Hashimoto's or non-Hashi's hypothyroid, it's common to discover problems in other parts of the body that need to be addressed--inadequate iron, vitamin D or B12, high cholesterol or blood pressure, iodine deficiency, etc.

Low Serum Iron (also called total iron)

As thyroid patients have been changing to a better treatment containing direct T3 like NDT or T4/T3, a large body have been surprised to discover they may have inadequate iron. And that in turn pushes RT3 up, which makes us more hypothyroid.

Causes of iron deficiency

1. Having a lowered metabolism from hypothyroid decreases the production of hydrochloric acid/stomach acid in your stomach, which in turn leads to a malabsorption of iron.
2. Continued hypothyroid also keeps your body temperature low, causing your body to make fewer red blood cells.
3. Additionally, in women, being hypothyroid can result in heavier periods, which causes more iron loss and less

storage iron.

The lower your iron levels, the faster your storage iron is used up. Though it's most common with women, men are not immune from having low iron.

Steph, who gave me her story, explains what happened her.

Like a few of my family members, I was put on levothyroxine. I expected to feel better. And I did at first. But the longer I was on it, I had to be honest with myself that there were problems that weren't going away, and new ones appearing. I was seeing more hair in the shower drain, my eyebrows were now thin, and I was having problems doing my job.

So thanks to STTM, I convinced my doctor to add T3 to my levo. And I raised it a few times to get where my free T3 should be. Except, I was feeling worse as I moved up in the range. Then, my mother pushed me to test my iron. And there it was. My iron was too low. Not only was that making me feel bad, but I later found out my RT3 was high. I started on iron and lowered my T4 a to help get the RT3 down. It took a few weeks, but I did start to feel better. And I got my iron where it should be.

The slide into low iron can be symptomless at first, but it eventually becomes the precursor to being anemic as your hemoglobin levels fall in your blood, which are the molecules in your blood which transport oxygen to your tissues. And once the latter occurs, you can become easily breathless.

The move from declining iron into anemia causes symptoms so similar to being hypothyroid that many patients make the wrong conclusion that their desiccated thyroid or T3 is too low or not working. Excessively low iron can also make it difficult to continue raising your desiccated thyroid or T4/T3!

Biologically, insufficient iron levels may be affecting the first two of three steps of thyroid hormone formation by reducing the activity of the enzyme thyroid peroxidase, which is dependent on iron. Iron deficiency, in turn, may also alter thyroid metabolism and reduce the conversion of T4 to T3, besides modifying the binding of T3, i.e. making a certain amount of T3 unusable. Low iron can produce too-high levels of RT3. Additionally, low iron levels can increase circulating concentrations of TSH (thyroid stimulating hormone). Iron, in addition to iodine, selenium and zinc, is essential for normal thyroid hormone metabolism.

Symptoms of low iron

Low iron mimics the hypothyroid state, and depending on your individual symptoms, can include depression, achiness, easy fatigue, weakness, feeling cold, faster heart rate, palpitations, loss of sex drive, foggy thinking, and breathlessness on exertion, etc. I personally found it hard to even climb the stairs in my house, and noted excess burning in my legs from a build-up of lactic acid. That has always been a key sign for me that my iron is now too low!

Why you need four labs related to iron

Here are four labs we learned that are needed when it comes to iron:
- **Serum iron** (also called total iron)
- **% saturation**
- **TIBC** (we don't usually need UIBC)
- **Ferritin**

Serum iron: This is measuring the amount of your circulating iron that is bound to the protein called transferrin—the latter which carries iron around. Up to 90% of your total iron is bound to the protein transferrin which carries the iron around. For **women,** optimal serum iron seems to get this "close to" 110 in broad ranges that are similar to 27-159, or 50-180, give or take. Some ranges just go up to 30ish, give or take, and optimal serum iron for women seems to be "around" 23 . For **men,** optimal in the broad range is usually in the 130's, and in smaller ranges that end around 30ish, close to the top.

% Saturation: We see this "close to or at" 35% (or. 35) for *women* when their iron is optimal, or "close to or at" 38% (or .38) for *men* when their iron is optimal. The percentage represents what is being occupied by iron in the iron-binding

sites of transferrin.

TIBC: This stands for "total iron binding capacity" and is an indirect measure of whether your liver is making enough of the protein called transferrin, which is meant to bind to the iron and carry it around through your body like a taxi. If the range is "around" 250 to 450 or so, this should be in the lower 300's (or lower) when you have enough serum iron.

Some of us remain in the 200's somewhere no matter what, so we have to take the protein lactoferrin (available on supplement websites or vitamin stores) when we are taking iron supplements, perhaps 1-2 capsules each time we take iron. Our low TIBC implies that the ability of transferrin to bind iron and carry it around is impaired for us. That is me.

When serum iron is too low, the TIBC usually is in the mid-300s or higher in those broader ranges (except in those of us with chronically low TIBC no matter what.)

Ferritin: This represents the protein that holds and stores our iron for future use, so it's also representing our storage iron. Note that is NOT a lab that you treat. What we treat is serum iron. We are looking at ferritin to discern inflammation mostly. It will go high when inflammation is a problem.

There is usually a broad range for ferritin. And for women, when serum iron is too low, ferritin will be 50's or below. When serum iron is optimal, this will be higher than the 50's in most cases, and up to 70-90 depending on the individual for **women**. For **men**, optimal ferritin seems to be in the 110's.

mine was 72

> *If ferritin is high (above the 90s for **women**; 120's or higher for **men**), that represents that you have inflammation. The body wisely thrusts iron into storage, since that very iron can feed inflammation.*

But the higher ferritin goes, the potentially worse one's inflammation is. And high inflammation can be dangerous. So we need to get it down by finding the cause of the inflammation, and/or getting inflammation down. Both.

Hashimoto's patients can have high inflammation due to

the attack on the thyroid, made worse by eating gluten, other foods, infections, or having high stress. Non-Hashi's patients can have inflammation just due to being poorly treated. Until we figure out the cause of our inflammation and turn it around, taking anti-inflammatories is a good thing! They include, but are not limited to, curcumin, fish oil, cat's claw, rose hips, and more. Any good vitamin/health food store can have great mixtures of anti-inflammatory supplements to explore. If inflammation is especially serious, talk to your doctor about a prescription anti-inflammatory.

Other labs to confirm inflammation

Every once in a while, the ferritin lab doesn't confirm inflammation in an individual, even if for the majority, it does. So this is where you get two other labs: C-Reactive Protein test (CRP) as well as the Erythrocyte Sedimentation Rate test (ESR) or the White Blood Count (WBC).

Lab example of why ferritin isn't enough information

When this patient got her lab results back, she found out why the ferritin isn't enough. You will note that her ferritin result is perfect---between 70 and 90 is the goal for a female. But her serum levels and saturation were far too low, revealing her ferritin level had risen in response to inflammation.

- **Ferritin:** 82
- **Iron, Serum:** 49 (range was 35-155, and result should be "around" 110)
- **Iron Saturation:** 18 (range was 17-55, and result should be "close to" 35% for women)
- **TIBC:** 333 (range was 250-370, and is a bit high.

How to prepare for iron testing

At the minimum, the Iron Institute recommends to be off iron supplementation for up to five days to see what you are holding onto.

The solution to having low iron

Once you have verified low iron with a blood test, the next step is to supplement. Yes, we can also incorporate high iron foods in our diet. But it usually isn't enough to get those low levels up. So we look at iron supplementation. And remember: you have to have treated inflammation for this to work.

Kinds of Iron Supplements

There are a large variety of iron supplements. Some are **Ferrous Sulfate, Ferrous Glutamate, Ferrous Fumarate**, etc. *Ferrous Sulfate* is usually the cheapest, and some patients add Vitamin E to their supplementation since Ferrous Sulfate may slightly deplete levels of Vitamin E. *But it's very prone to making us constipated.*

Ferrous Gluconate and *Ferrous Fumarate* may cause fewer symptoms, and both are milder on the stomach and absorb well. But again, they can be prone to making us constipated.

Ferrous Bisglycinate, a chelated amino acid iron supplement which can be easy to tolerate, is one that is much less likely to make us constipated!! I personally always use this version when I need to move my iron up to optimal.

Liquid iron is a good choice if you use the vegetable-based (non-heme) type. Beware of liquid iron that is animal based (heme)–it can temporarily blacken your teeth, as it did to my bottom teeth. The right liquid iron is very absorbable, and you might be able to take slightly less than I mentioned in the next heading.

Food-based iron tablets can work, but again, you have to see how much iron is in it in order to take enough to get iron up. We are also forced to check all ingredients in any food-based iron product, as by taking enough tablets to get our iron up, we are also raising whatever else is in it. The next heading explains how much iron we take to get our levels up.

Grass-fed beef liver supplements have iron in them as well as well many other nutrients, such as phosphorus, potassium, vitamin A, biotin, folate and more...but the copper content is high. And that can be a problem unless you have very good levels of zinc to counter the copper.

It's recommended to take Vitamin C with your iron supplementation, which helps the absorption of iron and counters free radicals produced by iron. At the very least, drink down your iron tablets with orange juice or a Vitamin C rich drink. Also taking a mineral supplement can assist the absorption, as can B-vitamins with an emphasis on B6.

Avoid excess soy (which you should be doing anyway as a thyroid patient) which decreases absorption of iron, as does black tea, zinc, calcium, high fiber, and even eating excess egg yolks. Use moderation in any of these foods, supplements or liquids if your iron is low.

How much iron supplementation we take

It's important to read the label of any kind of iron you take to discover how much *"elemental iron"* is in each tablet. That's the total amount of iron that is absorbable in any particular supplement. Iron bisglycinate shows it directly by the milligram (mg) they list on the label. Others will show a high mg amount, yet the elemental iron content is quite low. Read the label!!

Hypothyroid patients have discovered it can take up to **150 - 200 mg total daily of "elemental iron"** daily, split and taken with meals to prevent stomach upset, to help raise their low iron. And it can take up to eight weeks minimum to get it up. Thus many of us retest our iron (after being off up to 5 days) in about 4-6 weeks to see our progress.

Do I need an iron infusion?

There are some patients whose iron is so very low that their doctor does recommend an IV iron infusion. You are usually monitored to prevent the rare anaphylactic shock. But be aware if you have inflammation, as that will push a lot of that iron into storage, aka ferritin, and doctors often seem to forget about this. So getting that inflammation down can be crucial. There are also prescription anti-inflammatory medications.

Dealing with inconvenient side effects of our iron supplementation

Taking certain iron supplements can cause constipation or small round stools. Taking a good magnesium supplement can be a wise counter, taken twice a day, until you find the amount that softens your stools. There are also prescription laxatives that can help and are safer for longer use.

Since iron can bind thyroid hormones, patients have learned to take their NDT, T4/T3 or T3 away from the iron, such as 2-4 hours.

When iron levels are back up

Several patients have found out the hard way that their iron levels can plummet all over again if they are still hypothyroid. So until we get out of our hypothyroid state, it may be wise to stick with a small dose of supplemental iron and/or eat iron rich foods, especially if you are female and still menstruating. Once into menopause, your iron levels may stay where they need to.

Thalassemia and Polycythemia Vera

It's important to mention that there are some uncommon conditions that cannot be corrected by taking iron: Thalassemia and Polycythemia Vera. With Thalassemia, an inherited condition causing your body to make an abnormal form of oxygen-carrying hemoglobin, iron supplementation can cause an iron overload because of the missing gene in your hemoglobin. Blood transfusions can be necessary. Polycythemia Vera equates to having too many red blood cells, making your blood really thick. If your hemoglobin and hematocrit lab results are high, you'll want your doctor to check for the above conditions.

Vitamin B-12 deficiency

B12 is an essential vitamin for the health of your red blood cells and your nervous system, as well as the creation of DNA and cell division. It's mainly found in meat, poultry and fish, plus milk products and eggs.

B12 is released in your stomach by hydrochloric acid. Yet, because hypothyroid can result in low levels of hydrochloric acid / stomach acid, having a low level of vitamin B12 can go hand-in-hand with .

Stress can also lower B12 levels. So it can be wise to have your B12 levels tested, especially since the deficiency of B12 is gradual, and it can be more severe than your symptoms reveal.

When symptoms finally show themselves, they can include weakness and fatigue, confusion, balance problems, bruising, and paleness, as well as shortness of breath, feeling dizzy and a rapid heart rate. Later stages can result in a tingling in your extremities, called neuropathy, or a red irritated tongue and loss of taste.

> *I personally know my B12 is too low when my fingers can go to sleep easily, or my legs when I'm in a hard chair, or on the floor sitting cross-legged.*

John Dommisse, MD of Tucson, AZ, in the article titled *Hidden Causes of Dementia*, feels that the "normal ranges" for B12 deficiencies start out way too low. And we agree!!

Ranges for B12 considered "normal" will vary from country to country. **Generally, we discovered that we need to be in the upper quarter of any range to get rid of lingering symptoms of low B12. Years of experiences on that!**

There are different B12 varieties:

- **Methylcobalamin**, the active form of B12
- **Adenosylcobalamin**, another active form of B12 which works with our mitochondria and ATP to make energy
- **Hydroxycobalamin,** a precursor form of vitamin B_{12} which converts to both methylcobalamin and adenosylcobalamin.
- **Cyanocobalamin,** a manmade form of B12

Many patients prefer the methyl- version. I personally take the Adenosyl- version with Hydroxy-.

Another more serious form of vitamin B-12 deficiency is called Pernicious Anemia, which is an autoimmune disorder and can be paired for some patients who have Hashimoto's

Thyroiditis, another autoimmune problem. Just as with a normal deficiency, your body is unable to absorb the B-12 from your digestive tract. Treatment consists of the tablets or injections.

> *Do all patients who have low B12 (but do not have autoimmune Pernicious Anemia), strongly need B12 injections?? Absolutely not. Most do great on just supplements. And many take 5000 mcg a day of B12 until they have built their levels back up.*

Having a Methylation problem due to the MTHFR or other mutations

From 2003 until today, there has been growing and interesting information about our genes. And a biggie is the MTHFR gene, aka this mouthful: *methylenetetrahydrofolate reductase*. The MTHFR gene mutation locations which can affect us the most are termed as C677T and A1298C.

How do we get mutations? From our parents. For example, if there's one mutation, it is passed down from one parent, called a *heterozygous mutation*. If there are two mutations, both parents passed them down, called a *homozygous mutation*. Risks of problems are higher with two, or one for 677 and one for 1298—the latter called *compound heterozygous*.

Those MTHFR mutations when active, especially 677, can raise the risk of one or more of the following for thyroid patients:

1. Folic acid not being able to convert to the active form called methylfolate, or high levels of folate
2. Homocysteine to build up in the blood, causing problems
3. B12 to build high in the blood, causing a low B12 state
4. Metals being high in the blood
5. Cardiovascular or stroke risk
6. Increased risk of cancers
7. Increased risk of miscarriages

Finding oneself with high B12 is especially common for thyroid patients with an active MTHFR mutation—a methylation problem. It results in a low B12 state.

What a methylation problem can do to iron

One sure-fire way to know we have a methylation problem is seeing a low ferritin with a good or high iron. Or, if serum iron looks optimal or high with a high TIBC, another clue.

Testing for mutations

For one, *www.23andme.com* can reveal them after the raw data is uploaded to *livewello.com*. You might also get testing from your doctor.

How to treat this mutation

Dr. Ben Lynch feels that "repairing the digestive system and optimizing the flora should be one of the first steps in correcting methylation deficiency", and that especially includes treating candida because of the toxins it releases, inhibiting proper methylation.[22]

Here's an excellent page about treating MTHFR: *https:// blog.bulletproof.com/the-mthfr-gene-mutation-and-how-to-rewire-your-genetics/* (If the URL eventually changes, just do an internet search for "treatment of the mthfr gene)

There are other causes for a methylation problem, and I've already written a lot here to give more info: *http:// stopthethyroidmadness.com/mthfr*

High Cholesterol

Remarkably, a large percentage of hypothyroid patients, especially those who remain on the inadequate T4-only treatment, have rising or high cholesterol. And sadly, the typical approach by their doctors is to see it as a separate condition from their hypothyroid.

Cholesterol is a soft yet waxy substance that hangs out with the fats in your bloodstream and is also found in your tissue and cells. And cholesterol is the substance from which estrogen, progesterone, testosterone, DHEA and cortisol are made. So cholesterol is positively essential for your balanced health.

---

[22] https://www.thedailybeast.com/how-to-rewire-your-genetics-hacking-the-mthfr-gene-mutation

But with hypothyroidism, cholesterol may not be adequately metabolized, resulting in an unhealthy buildup. And you can have a higher triglyceride level and low HDL– the good cholesterol. The result is an increased risk for cardiovascular disease and a doctor who wants to put you on statin medications which are problematic in themselves, potentially causing memory problems, muscle weakness, and peripheral neuropathy.

The solution is to treat your hypothyroid with desiccated thyroid or T3 and dose until *optimal*, seeking a high range free T3. Remember, though, that we have to have the right amount of cortisol to achieve this without problems.

Iodine deficiency

When patients chat in thyroid groups, it's not uncommon to see them ponder why there is such an explosion of hypothyroid problems worldwide. We know there can be many causes, and one in particular is iodine-deficient soils from which some food is grown. In addition, the amount toxins we are all exposed to in our environment, including fluoride, bromide, chloride, chlorine and mercury, compete with iodine for the same cell receptors, which can result in many us having low iodine.

And since one of the primary functions of iodine in your body is the formation of thyroid hormones, low iodine can be serious. It also plays a role in the health of your heart, brain, female hormones, breast health, and immune system.

One of my favorite books on the subject of breast health is *Breast Cancer and Iodine: How to Prevent and How to Survive Breast Cancer* by David Derry, MD.

In most cases, your greatest intake of dietary iodine comes from refined table salt. But is it enough? In your diet, iodine can be quite variable depending on the amount of iodized in the food product, or the feed of the animal eaten. With the growing interest by patients in sea salt, which is usually not iodized, the levels of dietary iodine .

Testing your iodine levels

It's very important to find out if you need iodine or not.

Considered the most accurate assessment of your iodine levels is the "iodine loading test", which is measuring the excretion of your iodine over a 24-hour time frame. The lower the excretion of iodine, the greater likelihood of low iodine levels. You swallow a total of 50 mg of an Iodoral tablet. Then in the next 24 hours, you collect your urine to be sent in for analysis. Iodine labs include: FFP Laboratories, whose email is: *ffp_lab@ yahoo.com* or Doctors Data, Inc at *www.doctorsdata.com* Or you can do one via LabCorp or Quest Diagnostics.

Author Lynne Farrow has written a very well-received book titled *The Iodine Crisis: What You Don't Know About Iodine Can Wreck Your Life,* which is also sold on Amazon.

Supplementing with iodine

Iodine supplementation has grown in popularity, especially with thyroid patients when they find themselves low after testing. The most popular supplements are Iodoral in pill form, 12.5 mgs & 50 mgs, or Lugols, 2% or 5% as a liquid added to your favorite juice. One drop of 5% Lugols has approximately 6.25 mg of iodine (plus 3-4 mg potassium).

Recommended doses are up to 50 mg, but some Hashimoto's patients often find it important to go much lower, and raise slower, as the detox can make things worse. Most avoid taking it after the afternoon, since iodine intake in the evenings can keep you awake.

Side effects with iodine

If the iodine loading test reveals you are low, you'll need to know that the use of iodine acts as a detoxing agent, especially against excess bromide, fluoride and chloride. So be prepared for potential side effects like fatigue, pimples, headaches, etc. They will eventually go away, and it helps to take companion nutrients to counter those side effects, which includes vitamin C, B-vitamins, vitamin D, and minerals like selenium, magnesium and zinc. You can also take smaller amounts of iodine and only slowly build up, if needed.

It's also helpful to keep all of your detox pathways open. Many teas can help do that, like dandelion, lemon and ginger, nettle and chamomile. The herb milk thistle seeds is known to help with your liver and detoxing, though you'll need to take iron with it, as milk thistle can lower iron.

Iodine and Hashimoto's

Turns out there can be two opposite sides of the coin for Hashimoto's patients and iodine use. Some Hashimoto's patients find iodine to exacerbate their autoimmune symptoms and make them feel far worse. That's probably due to the detox iodine causes, thus the importance to prepare and go low and slow.

Others have been very pleased to find out iodine outright lowered their antibodies!

Iodine and stressed adrenals

There is concern by some adrenal patients that either the toxin release caused by iodine, or the improvement of thyroid function with iodine, further stressed their adrenals. That can be a reality as experienced and reported by some adrenal patients.

Other the other side of the coin, there are others with adrenal fatigue who found the iodine-caused toxin release not being a problem at all if they were taking certain supporting, companion nutrients along with the iodine.

Victoria, an adrenal dysfunction patient, relates the following example of how those nutrients made a difference:

I was treated for adrenal exhaustion by an Integrative Medicine MD, without iodine for most of a year (she said my saliva test was the worst she'd ever seen). Nothing she did healed my situation, including adding 3mg of iodine/day-- just a minimal change. I then lost my insurance and couldn't consult with her anymore. After a crash in my health, I found out more about iodine) and learned about the whole protocol: higher amounts of iodine and most importantly, with companion nutrients plus additional supplements for healing adrenals. I took extra unrefined salt (1+ tablespoon per day), extra Vit C, Vit E (1200iu/day), started Vit D3 every day (8000iu), plus adrenal cortex

*(1-2 tabs per day) and pregnenolone (40-50 mg/day). After
2-3 months of this, I had to stop the adrenal cortex because
when I would take it, I would become over-adrenalated.
Since then, I can do my work for hours at a time and
not crash constantly. I have energy to spare and have been
doing music and performance with my partner and more.
Can go out and dance for hours. And also since then, have
lost at least 20 pounds and not regaining.*

Jody has found the use of iodine to be huge in confronting
her Hashimoto's:

*I heard about the use of iodine but was afraid of it, since
I read of problems if you use it with Hashimoto's. But I also
tested low when I did the iodine loading test, so I decided
to give it a try. I made sure I took plenty of selenium and
minerals with salt water. I started low and built up. After
two months, I noticed that my heart palps had ceased.
Four months after I started, my doctor agreed to test my
antibodies. Both were lower! I was shocked. And they have
continued to fall. I also lost all sign of my fibrocystic breast
disease.*

All of this is going to be an individual call. Some avoid iodine
altogether with adrenal dysfunction so as not to make it worse:
others take a *much lower dose* than 50 mg, such as 12.5, and do
well. I personally am in the latter amount. Others, like Victoria,
find success with iodine and adrenal fatigue if they are taking
supporting nutrients and detox teas or herbs.

Because iodine use can be a controversial subject with
adrenal dysfunction, I encourage you to join good iodine social
media group and seek opinions before deciding what is best
for you. An excellent book on the subject is *Iodine: Why You
Need It, Why You Can't Live Without It* (3nd Edition) by David
Brownstein, MD.

Hypopituitary

Hypopituitarism is about a poorly-functioning pituitary
gland which results in a sluggish release (or no release) of

certain messenger hormones...like the TSH. The most common cause is having an adenoma—a benign tumor on the gland. It's detected by a scan. Causes include whiplash of your neck (such as if someone hits your car from behind), or a problem in the hypothalamus, which messages the pituitary.

When healthy, your pituitary secretes messenger hormones which direct the functioning of your thyroid, adrenals, or sex hormones. For the thyroid, that hormone is the TSH (thyroid stimulating hormone), and for the adrenals, it's the ACTH. A good clue of hypopituitary, along with symptoms of fatigue, feeling cold, depression, low blood pressure, etc. is having a very low TSH lab result along with a low free T3. You can also have a low ACTH (Adrenocorticotropic hormone), low LH (Luteinizing hormone), low GH (growth hormone) and low FSH (follicle-stimulating hormone). So by testing pituitary messenger hormones, more clues result for hypopituitary when other messenger hormones are low.

Treatment for hypopituitary is the same as treatment for one's hypothyroidism, or low cortisol, or other hormones, as well as sex hormone treatment. Is it curable? Many will say no. Yet, we have seen one patient rid himself of his hypopituitary with the correct thyroid and adrenals treatment. Otherwise, it can be for life.

Thyroid Cancer (Thyca)

There's nothing more shocking to find out you have thyroid cancer. Some patients diagnosed with it weren't even aware it existed, and definitely didn't expect it in themselves. And women are three times more likely to develop it than men.

In the early stages, there can be no symptoms of thyroid cancer. Later, it's usually discovered when a nodule is found on the thyroid by touch, viewed with an ultrasound, and cancer confirmed after doing a fine needle biopsy. (Luckily, medical articles state that only 1-5% of those nodules are cancerous, i.e. just because you find a nodule doesn't mean you have cancer.) Other symptoms of cancer in the thyroid can include cough or hoarseness, swelling of your neck or difficulty swallowing, but these can also be from Hashimoto's disease.

What causes it? There appears to be multiple higher-risk possibilities. Excess radiation exposure is one known risk, such as from repeated x-ray treatments for acne, dental x-rays, etc. Radioactive fallout is another risk, such as the Chernobyl accident in 1986, or the nuclear reactor meltdown in Japan in 2011. Genetics can increase your risk due to an altered gene. Low iodine raises the risk of thyroid cancer. Some patients who find themselves with thyroid cancer have none of the above risks.

A lab test to help confirm cancer, especially papillary and follicular (see below), is called Tg, or Thyroglobulin, which might be made by thyroid cancer cells. Note: if you test positive for antibodies against thyroglobulin (which are antibodies used to diagnose Hashimoto's disease), your Tg will not be a reliable tumor marker for thyroid cancer, says research.

There are four basic forms of thyroid cancer:

- **Papillary** *(which are the majority of cases, related to radiation exposure, highly curable),*
- **Follicular** *(more aggressive, seen in iodine deficiency)*
- **Medullary** *(in the parafollicular cells which make calcitonin*
- **Anaplastic** *(least common, very malignant).*

Most cancers of the thyroid are treated via removal of the lobe which contained the cancer, and often the other side in many cases. Radioactive iodine (RAI) is a conventional, even if controversial, follow-up treatment, since thyroid cells continue to absorb iodine, and the excess iodine becomes a form of chemotherapy. Alternative practitioners can use holistic treatments to ease side effects caused by needed conventional treatments of thyroid cancer. The latter would be important to talk about with a good doctor.

Thyca is a non-profit organization for thyroid cancer survivors with lots of great information for you: *http://thyca.org.*

WARNING: most surgeons/doctors will tend to put you on T4-only after thyroid removal. They simply have poor understanding that putting you on simply a storage hormone is the worst way to treat one's now-hypo state. Instead, we can need T3, and then switch to NDT.

ODDS AND ENDS TIDBITS

* If inflammation is driving your ferritin up, curcumin with Meriva has proven to be an excellent treatment in higher amounts than what is recommended on the bottle. More supplements are mentioned here: http://stopthethyroidmadness.com/inflammation

* Iodine proponents underscore the use of iodine supplementation to prevent thyroid cancer from radiation in the environment.

* Some patients have reported seeing their thyroid nodules disappear with the use of iodine and NDT.

* Working on everything and still seem to have problems? Time to ask your doctor about testing your EBV (Epstein Barr Virus) levels, other viruses and bacteria, plus Lyme disease.

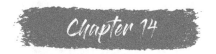

Chapter 14

PATIENTS HAVE A STORY TO TELL

E ven with all the ground-breaking information in this book, the most inspiring part can be the stories of others who have lived it. Here are a few to inspire you, and there are millions more across the world. Note that some of these stories refer to the natural desiccated thyroid. But many also find success with T4/T3.

Meleese Pollock's story:

My story starts in 1994, when I not only started to feel fatigued, but also my mind, numbingly so. I had gained 23 kilos and I had never had a weight problem in my life.

And the fatigue!!! I would go to bed at night and *die* with 10 - 11 hours of sleep as if I'd been doped up. Then I would drag myself out of bed and stand in the kitchen and cry because I was too tired to get the children out of bed and ready for school.

I had my three children when I was 28, 35 and 38 years old. I finally went to the doctor who thank goodness tested my thyroid function, I had the answer! I was diagnosed with Hashi's/hypo- and prescribed Oroxine (the Australian brand for synthetic T4) 100 mcg. After 3 months I was re-tested and it was increased to 150 mcg. Over the next couple of years, I had 2 further increases–first to 200 mcg, then 300 mcg–the latter where I stayed for the next 10 years. And yet, I still had crippling fatigue. I couldn't lose the weight and had major depression.

I got on the internet, started searching for answers and learned about Natural Desiccated Thyroid (NDT). I had first heard about it from a naturopath who had called it "pig thyroid". I found that here in Australia, I could get compounded capsules made up with imported thyroid USP. The compounding chemist said that I need 180 mg (3 grains) as that was equivalent to 300 mcg Oroxine.

So I started the compounded natural thyroid and within a few days felt better. I had blood tests done at around 3 months and was horrified to find that my TSH had shot up to over 6.

So I went back on Oroxine. I simply thought NDT wasn't working for me, was doing something wrong and it was my fault. Things continued to go downhill for me. I decided I was going to end my life if things hadn't improved. And all of this occurred while having a TSH of 0.05, a Free T3 of 5.2 with 5.3 at the upper end of the range, and a Free T4 of 19 with an upper range of 23. Perfect labs and still all the symptoms!!

About 18 months ago, I decided to give the desiccated thyroid one more shot after I found out that you dose by symptoms *and the frees*, not to a "conversion formula". I have slowly worked my way up to what seems to be my optimal dose of 390 mg (6 and ½ grains is optimal for me) I cannot believe the difference! My energy levels are so much better, the brain fog/depression is going and... drum roll...I have lost 23 kilos! (about 50 pounds). NDT has saved my life

Nancy Kay Adam's story:

It almost brings me to tears to write my story, but I want to contribute. I have been a runner since high school. I competed in many meets and won a lot of them. I was also good at tennis.

In college, I continued with it and also had many accomplishments. I've got a lot of ribbons and trophies in my display cabinet which I'm proud of.

When I got out of college, I got married to my sweetheart, and we immediately had Michael. And I think that's where this all began. I just didn't feel right after he was born, and I could not lose that extra poundage. 15 months later, I had Emily. And it was even worse this time. I was really tired, and had post-partum depression. And I was getting very pudgy, which bothered me greatly.

I thought I could work it off by running again, which I tried. The high school nearby had a great track I could use. But I was wrong. Each time I went, I was become more tired than ever. I just crossed it all off to being a young mother.

Fast forward 5 more years, and I had gained even more weight! I couldn't run, and my doctor kept telling me my problem was eating too much and exercising too little, since everything he tested came back normal! I was also now on an anti-depressant. But I'll tell you, I was still really depressed.

And I was also starting to feel a lot of anxiety. Sure, I loved my kids and being their mom, and we were in a gorgeous house thanks to my husband's new job. But I looked horrible and felt as bad. Those were bad years in spite of all the good.

Finally, I met Janie while sitting beside each other at an outdoor violin concert. And as we got to know each other better, she gave me some information that I found quite curious. I did the reading that she told me to do, and made an appointment with a doctor about 2 hours away that she recommended.

To make a long story short, I found out I was hypothyroid all this time, that the TSH wasn't telling it at all, and that I had the beginning of adrenal fatigue. I started on adrenal cortex, and later switched to prescription HC (hydrocortisone). I needed to be on desiccated thyroid, which I did with this new doctor after she helped me raise the HC. I had few bumps–had to tell her that I wanted to keep raising from where she thought I should stay. And now, I feel 100% better. 100% percent. I'm already weaned down my HC, and I've started running again, too. This is wonderful.

Helen Trimble's story:

After months of a rapid decline in my health, accompanied by an endless list of terrifying symptoms, the diagnosis of hypothyroidism and ensuing prescription of Synthroid gave me immediate psychological relief. I felt positive Synthroid would end the troublesome loss of muscle, hair and eyebrows, dry scaly skin, hoarse throat, debilitating fatigue, shortness of breath, restless legs, and incessant tingling of extremities.

It did not. I continued to regress further into a deep, dark funk and was severely depressed. I lost the ability to think clearly; needed a cane to walk; suffered from sleepless, unbearable pain-filled nights, experienced incessant loss of breath, nighttime seizures; horrific heart palpitations and continued loss of hair. Synthroid was sending me to my grave. I was literally dying and contemplated suicide. My physical and mental deterioration were just too great to bear. I was no longer terrified of death; I was now afraid of living. I realized that I was no longer good for anyone and was soon going to be another poorly treated thyroid statistic.

According to my doctor, the labs were normal. *"Normal?,"* I asked. *"How can you sit there and tell me I am normal when I look and walk like this?"*

She had no reply. She just shrugged her shoulders. I told my doctor that I wanted to try desiccated thyroid. She protested, but finally agreed. I was in such bad shape that a new prescription was worth a try.

Within two weeks, my deteriorating mind, body and spirit was rapidly changing for the better, and into week four, I was able to walk without the aid of a cane and the muscle pain and cramping was gone. I began to sleep soundly, the shortness of breath and heart palpitations stopped, and I developed wonderful tufts of new hair growth on my scalp along with the reappearance of long-lost eyebrows. Throughout the day, I had renewed energy and the brain fog was a thing of the past. Further blood test showed I was anemic, and I started ferritin supplementation and supplementation and B12 shots. In a few months, the fatigue disappeared.

Switching from Synthroid to NDT saved me from suicide

and a life of disability. NDT stopped the thyroid madness I was experiencing and brought balance back to my life. Today, I am working full time, completing my Master's degree from the University of Phoenix, and living life to the fullest.

Kerry Bergus' story:

About the time I started into puberty, my mother, who was an RN, began to think I had hypothyroid problems, in spite of always having "normal" results when an endocrinologist would check my thyroid levels. My periods were so heavy and painful that I had to stay home from school a few days each month and live on codeine.

I was finally put on birth control pills. My breasts grew huge, from a B cup to a D cup almost overnight. My periods were no longer painful or heavy, but I began to have great anxiety with no reason. I gained some weight in spite of being active with drum corps and other activities. After high school, I went off the birth control pills and began to have horrible sebaceous acne. I also put on weight and the painful heavy periods returned.

In my late teens and into my twentieth year, chronic tonsillitis and sinus infections resulted in the removal of my tonsils when I was 21. I was depressed and considered suicide seriously once. Thankfully my mother saved me from myself. From that point on, I struggled with major anxiety and bouts of depression with thoughts of suicide from time to time. In my late twenties I married and began my journey in to motherhood. After my first child was born, I lost the baby weight within six weeks and was happily in my pre-pregnancy jeans. Within six months I was pregnant again, but this time, the weight didn't come off after the second birth. My muscle tone deteriorated, my hair fell out and I felt tired most of the time. My dry and flaky skin resembled a snake and the anxiety increased.

When we wanted a third child a couple of years later, we struggled with fertility. When I finally got pregnant, it was difficult. My weight climbed, though my eating didn't change. I was very sick with diarrhea throughout; my hair fell out and I ended up with high blood pressure. Post-delivery, my weight didn't drop despite eating less, my hair continued to fall out and my blood pressure stayed high. I ended up having an endometrial ablation to stop the hemorrhage type bleeding with each period.

As the years went by, my weight climbed, hair stayed thin and my marriage deteriorated. When I became a single mom, I was diagnosed with low thyroid and my OB-Gyn put me on Synthroid. I noticed no difference in the way I felt, even with increases. He would check my TSH, and then declare I was fine. An endocrinologist then declared that I had Hashimoto's autoimmune thyroiditis. By this time my cholesterol was 217 and I felt lousy.

I knew that I needed something more and so began searching the internet, where I found a natural thyroid hormone group—Janie's. I finally found a group that knew exactly what I was going through. The women were so supportive and insightful that it was like receiving a cup of cold water on a hot day. I finally went to my doctor and asked her to change me from Synthroid to NDT. She had never heard of NDT, but agreed to write me a prescription.

As I made my way up to 3 grains, we saw dramatic changes in my cholesterol, down from 217 to 139. My skin became so soft and supple that I hardly ever use lotion anymore. No more acne breakouts and a reduction in blood pressure medication. All of this was due to my change from Synthroid to NDT. My life has improved so much and my energy has returned. The anxiety that I lived with for over thirty years has completely resolved. I thought I would have to live with it forever and NDT has given me my life back.

T.F.'s story:

For years, my wife told me I'm a typical man, because I refused to go to the doctor. But when my problems finally added up and even affected my work (I own a golfing store), I went. I was finally tired of being tired and out of breath. And my wife wasn't too turned on by my girth. Turns out that I had a bad back (which I obviously knew), and I'm hypo-. So the doc put me on Levoxyl. I think it kinda helped, but it didn't either. I was still tired and my back hurt.

About two years later, my wife, who is an internet buff, told me about NDT. I said okay and talked to my doc. He's actually my neighbor and my wife had to prod him. But I finally got switched. It definitely has made a difference. I've also found out that my iron levels weren't too swift, so am working on that, too. I'm impressed. You don't hear about men much with hypothyroid, but I did, and I've met a few others now who have it. NDT has really worked. My back has even improved because I can use our treadmill in the basement now.

Cathy's story:

We had severe and ongoing stress for years with the death of my father and the theft of my husband's machines and tools for his livelihood. It continued with his also getting a severe hernia and having surgery. Continuing on, we had problems with our oldest two children, affecting our youngest child in a negative way. Then our house burned down and we found we were $100,000 under-insured. Our stress levels soared as the problems with the neighborhood druggies more and more affected our older two children. This went on for a number of years until they left home.

My Chiro told me I was adrenally-challenged in the early part of this century, around 2000 - 2001, but I didn't have a clue as to what that meant so I pretty much ignored what he said. But I was steadily getting sicker and more hypo- and the docs would only give me Synthroid. I did some online research and discovered NDT, but couldn't find a doc to prescribe it. I was ill and desperate in 2005 - 2006 and found the Yahoo thyroid groups and finally found support. I initially started NDT and then read that adrenal problems can compound hypo-problems, so discontinued NDT and got some adrenal cortex with my Chiro's blessing. I also started Iodoral (iodine) around then also, figuring that with my long history from childhood of hypo- symptoms that were undiagnosed that I was most probably also iodine deficient.

After I worked my way up to 3 - 4 or so adrenal cortex per day, I added the NDT back in and gradually increased the

Adrenal Cortex up to 8 - 10 per day, and also increasing the NDT in conjunction with the adrenal cortex until I was at 6.75 grains. I should mention that once I got to 8 - 10 adrenal cortex per day, I switched to HC at around 25 mg daily.

I did better than I did on syncrap, but something was still missing, so I investigated Reverse T3 and figured that with all the severe stress, and I do mean severe and ongoing, that RT3 was probably an issue. I did not have money for independent testing, so I put myself on a temporary trial of T3, which I am still on, trying to clear the receptors. Once I run out of T3, I will have been on it for approximately 3 - 4 months or so, at which time I will be switching back to NDT by swapping it out, and may keep a little T3 in the mix, depending on how things go. During this whole time my need for HC (prescription hydrocortisone) stayed steady for several months.

Gradually it seemed the amount of HC I was taking was too much as I would feel some hyper symptoms, so I reduced the dosage to 22.5 and held steady for several months. Once again it seemed like too much, so I pared it down to 17.5 mg daily and was there for a few months. During this time of reducing the dosage I was forgetting doses here and there, with no ill effects, which told me my need for HC was reduced. I felt shaky 2-3 times, but that is all, and I haven't stress dosed now for several days and am fine, so I conclude my need for HC on a daily and regular basis is now reduced until I was at 10 mg daily, then 5 mg and then none. I have stress dosed for the asthma attacks and resulting past. I am vigilant, however, and will stress dose if I need to as I fully realize my adrenal state is most probably still somewhat fragile; the shakiness during the illness told me that, and as I still have a good supply of HC I will follow my symptoms like I have and stress dose when needed; I do NOT want to go the way of adrenal fatigue ever again if I can help it.

Chapter 15

GOoD FOOD, GOoD SUPPLEMENTS

nformed and better-treated thyroid and adrenal patients love eating healthier foods and taking certain supplements on their road to better health. And for good reason. Many of us discovered that we have been low in so many important nutrients—minerals like potassium, sodium, magnesium, selenium and/or iron, plus vitamins like D, B12 and more. Both poor diets and poor digestion due to hypothyroidism have played roles. And we have needed help in several areas.

Foods: Certain foods like vegetables and fruits, especially when raw and uncooked, are nutritionally dense and provide important enzymes needed for digestion and optimal health. Organic foods are said to provide less pesticides and other toxins. Some patients choose to go without meats; others find meat/protein important.

Supplements: Outside of good quality foods, we have also turned to supplements. Some brands of supplements may be better quality than others. For example, we have read that food-based vitamins may have higher processing standards. On the other hand, some state that synthetic vitamins are really the same as natural, molecule to molecule. Additionally, some brands may make better digestible products than others based on the fillers.

Good consumer organizations have warned about buying the super-cheap off-brands which, when tested, had less of at least one nutrient than stated. Bottom line, it will be the responsibility of each individual to research and decide what they are most comfortable with.

Note that the following lists are not exhaustive--just representative of several foods and supplements that thyroid patients report eating or taking.

What about gluten in foods? The vast majority of Hashimoto's patients have discovered they have to avoid gluten to achieve better health and the lowering of antibodies, as well as avoiding certain triggering foods (for them) that cause their antibodies to go up.

I strongly recommend the book ***Hashimoto's: Taming the Beast,*** as you will find much information based on patient reports, as to what foods have been problematic, and how many learn to eat.

FOODS

Almonds: These nuts are high in protein as well as magnesium, potassium, Vitamins E and B2. They are also high in oxalates, which are tiny crystal-like molecules. Most of us have no problem with oxalates, as they are moved out by our stools. Others can see kidney stones or other problems if they are in excess. Moderation is key in enjoying these nutritious nuts.

Almond Flour: This is a healthy alternative to wheat flour and is gluten-free, high in fiber and protein, and low in digestible carbs. There are many good recipes on the net. (Pancakes: cup of almond flour, two eggs, ¼ cup sparkling water, 2 tablespoons coconut oil, ¼ tsp salt, and touch of sweetener) See info below about coconut flour.

Apple Cider Vinegar (ACV) unfiltered: Who would have guessed, but when this age-old remedy is added to our favorite juice or water (up to one tablespoon), it greatly improves digestion and the problem of low stomach acid (a common issue with thyroid patients who are poorly treated) and can even remove lactose intolerance or lower blood sugar. Do know that it should never be consuming straight! To see even more benefits, check out this website:
http://www.earthclinic.com/Remedies/acvinegar.html.

Apricots: Even dried, these are a great source of potassium, which can go low in thyroid or adrenal patients, and two apricots are roughly equivalent to one 99 mg potassium pill. *If you are sensitive to sulfur, dried fruits can have sulfur dioxide in them, used in the drying process.*

Asparagus: Lo and behold, turns out this veggie may have some cancer-fighting properties with its histones and glutathione. It's also a good source of B6 plus has magnesium and many more nutrients. I prefer it steamed at the most, or raw. Asparagus shoots need to be young for best taste.

Avocados: Called the perfect food all in one, avocados are a good source of Potassium, Vit. A and C and contain the healthy monounsaturated fat. *Avocados are high in copper, so if you already have high levels of copper, this is a food to avoid or stay low with.* Otherwise, a great food!

Blueberries: A top-notch low-glycemic fruit, blueberries can reduce inflammation that is common in hypothyroidism and adrenal issues, as well as lower certain cancer risks. Research reveals that they improve memory, can reduce blood sugar, and elevate mood. They are rich in vitamin C as well as antioxidant phytonutrients called anthocyanidins, which enhance the vitamin C effects. Potentially great for one's adrenals and thyroid. I am a big fan of blueberries for their antioxidant status!

Brazil Nuts: Turns out these nuts are a good natural source of selenium, but only those which were grown in selenium rich soil. Many articles suggest to consume no more than two a day to meet your selenium needs. Also stated to be anti-inflammatory, immune system supportive, and anti-anxietal.

Cauliflower: When grated, this veggie makes a great pizza crust, believe it or not. (1 cup cooked, riced cauliflower, an egg, cup grated mozzarella cheese, 1/2 tsp fennel and 1 tsp oregano. Combine, press into crust size on pan. Bake 450 for 20 or so minutes. Add pizza or alfredo sauce. Meats and veggies of your choice. Broil more mozzarella on top.) *It's a goitrogen, which can suppress thyroid function, so eat in moderation.*

Chocolate: :) Yes, believe it or not, there is repeated evidence that those chocolate bars, *in moderation*, with the higher amounts of cocoa/cacao (70% or higher), have excellent antioxidant qualities, besides promoting heart and brain health. But what about the sugar content? That's up to the individual. But there are bars with mostly stevia as the sweetener.

Coconut flour: From coconut meat/meal, this is another gluten-free alternative that's high in fiber, healthy fats and even protein, and also makes great pancakes, for one. It's a good "flour-type" alternative if you have issues with nuts like almond flour. Check out recipes on the internet and cookbooks. Since coconut flour is very absorbent, less is used as compared to almond flour. Or you can combine them in certain recipes.

Coconut Oil: Turns out there are a lot of health benefits from this milky-white, shortening-looking oil. Scientific research shows it to help with digestion, weight, diabetes, energy, Alzheimer's and so much more. See Oils below.

Coconut water (not coconut milk): Turns out this nutritious drink is pretty high in potassium and minerals—even higher than a banana. It does have natural sugar. Highly recommended by many.

Donuts: Just kidding. Don't we wish.

Eggs: Like other proteins, eggs are a good source of B-vitamins, especially riboflavin (B2), and the yolk is rich in Vitamin A, plus D. Powdered egg whites make good high-protein drinks, and some are flavored. Great food if you are insulin resistant.

Fish, poultry, meats: These are all good sources of protein and b-vitamins, with chicken and turkey coming in slightly higher in protein. And increasing your amount of daily protein while lowering your carb intake helps with weight loss or maintenance—a boon for thyroid patients.

Oils/Fats: It doesn't have to be coconut oil to get benefits. Other quality oils include extra virgin olive, avocado, grapeseed, MCT, and more.

Onions: The antioxidant onion is rich in good nutrients, including Vit C, potassium, copper, manganese and Vit. B6. They may help bring high blood pressure down a bit due to the sulfur they contain, say some patients.

Probiotic foods: These are foods which can supply and feed the important good bacteria in your gut, which are highly important for your health and immune system. They include Kefir (a fermented drink), Kombucha (a fermented black or green tea drink), Sauerkraut (shredded fermented cabbage), Yogurt (the plain varieties are best. Greek Yogurt is lowest in carbs.), pickles, Miso (a seasoning) and Kimchi (a Korean dish).

Pumpkin Seeds: For those who find their magnesium levels too low, pumpkin seeds are a good food source of magnesium as well as protein and zinc. Most all seeds are good for us if you tolerate them! I personally keep a supply of raw, green pumpkin seeds for my Greek yogurt.

Spinach: This is one great veggie, and it's a good source of zinc, niacin and Vit. A, C, E, and K, plus iron, magnesium, potassium... and more. Add spinach in a blender with your favorite low glycemic berries, cottage cheese, vanilla, stevia, water, etc. and enjoy as a healthy blended drink. *Note that spinach is high in oxalates, so if your levels are already too high, this is not the veggie for you except in moderation.*

Tomatoes: This 'fruit' used as a veggie is full of the antibiotic lycopene and contains Vit. A, C, K, potassium and iron. Sprinkle parmesan cheese on top and broil for a great treat. *Tomatoes are nightshades, which some people note causes an allergic reaction. Other nightshades, include peppers, potatoes and eggplants.*

Tomato Juice: This is my favorite way to give myself potassium, as one cup is equal to approximately 450-500 mg.

Vegetable drinks in the blender: For those who don't like their veggies, placing them in the blender with an apple and its high Vit. C is a great way to promote continued good adrenal and thyroid health. Great mixtures come from spinach leaves or collard greens, celery, carrots, cucumbers, asparagus and more. *You may have to increase thyroid meds* *a bit if you do this regularly to counter the goitrogenic effect of some of these veggies.*

Yogurt: This is a good natural way to introduce the good bacteria lactobacillus bulgaricus and streptococcus thermophilus into your digestion and body. Check the labels to make sure it's loaded with good bacteria. Greek Yogurt can have the lowest carbs.

SUPPLEMENTS
(If in any doubt, you can do blood testing for any of the below before supplementing.)

Acidophilus: Not only does this help with digestion, this is an excellent supplement for vaginal health, putting good bacteria back in, and protecting against bad bacteria and parasites. It also seems to boost immune system health. If patients are using compounded desiccated thyroid, they ask for powdered acidophilus as the filler rather than cellulose.

ALA (Alpha Lipoic Acid): This is a fatty acid and antioxidant that helps convert your blood sugar into energy, so diabetics love it. It also helps with peripheral neuropathy. An added benefit is that it appears to inhibit tumor growth. ALA in higher amounts may inhibit conversion of T4 to T3.

Ashwagandha: This adaptogen herb seems to counter stress and anxiety as well as supports the immune system against cancer and disease. It's used to support already healthy adrenals, not to replace cortisol for sluggish adrenals.

B-vitamins: It's stated that your need for the energy-giving, water-soluble B-vitamins increases as you get healthier on desiccated thyroid or T4/T3, so many thyroid patients look for B-vitamin supplementation. They support your higher metabolism, skin tone, immune system, improve your emotional health and are huge for the health of your adrenals.

B5: (Pantothenic Acid): This is called the anti-stress B-vitamin and along with Vitamin C, has a strong relationship with the adrenal cortex function, which is why you'll often hear it recommended by informed doctors when you are under stress.

B6: This is one of the longest studied B-vitamins and can go low with thyroid problems. It's needed for your serotonin levels, as well as the immune system and red cell formation.

B12: It is all too common for thyroid patients to go low in this important B-vitamin after just a few years of being untreated or undertreated, which can contribute to high RT3 production. Without enough B12, you can suffer from dementia, irritability or depression, or tingling and/ or numbness of your fingers and toes, problems in your walking gait, or eyesight problems... plus more.

Cinnamon: This spice now comes in capsule form, because thyroid patients who have diabetes discovered that cinnamon can lower blood glucose levels. It's not dramatic—20-30% according to clinical studies, but worth the improvement. Suggested amounts are 1 – 4 grams (the latter equals ½ teaspoon). *Going much higher isn't good for our liver, say some researchers, and can thin our blood too much. So it's about moderation. .*

Coenzyme Q10: This is found naturally in your mitochondria cells but can go low with long-term untreated or undertreated hypo-, as well as by aging. It helps with heart function and other muscles, plus is a good antioxidant. CoQ10 supports your energy levels. And as you age, taking the more available version is key, aka ubiquinol instead of ubiquinone

Cod Liver Oil: This superfood nutritional supplement is great for heart function. It has high levels of Omega 3, is high in vitamins A and D, and for some, eases arthritic pain. The high levels of D are important since so many thyroid patients go low in D.

Eleuthero (Siberian Ginseng): This is an herbal adaptogen that helps deal with stress and may help prevent the dive into adrenal dysfunction, which will require cortisol. It helps boost concentration and immune function, as well.

Fish Oil: Luckily, fish oil is now made with flavorings like lemon and cherry which make it more consumable. And the latter is important since fish oil is high in the beneficial

Omega 3's. It seems to have good effect against depression.

Folate: This is a more readily available form of B9 as compared to folic acid, and doesn't have risk with its buildup in the body as does folic acid. It's especially crucial with active MTHFR mutations, or those like me who have several B9 mutations. Folate is especially important for the breakdown of amino acids.

Ginger: When I used to be on the lousy T4-only, I had bad tendonitis and inflammation in my fingers. Taking herbal ginger powder in capsules took that away, just as desiccated thyroid did the same. But I still take ginger to this day, as it has so many beneficial properties which range from reducing arthritic pain, to healthy heart function and lowering cholesterol, as well as the prevention or management of diabetes.

Grape Seed Extract: Stated to be a very safe, effective bioflavonoid antioxidant which improves the linings of your arteries, many doctors prescribe it to clear out fatty vessels. It helps decrease allergic responses, improves blood pressure and heart function. And...tah dahh...it can reduce wrinkles, say some sources. :)

Iodine: Since we are consuming so many chemicals in our food and water, iodine receptors get clogged or iodine is leeched out of our bodies due to toxins like fluoride, bromide and chloride. Thus, many thyroid patients supplement with iodine, either the liquid Lugols or the pill form called Iodoral. See Chapter 13 about iodine.

Krill Oil: This marine oil is very rich in EPA, DHA and Omega 3, and it does a good job of lowering inflammation. About 1000-2000 mg does the trick daily, say experts. *If you are allergic to shellfish, there may be concern.*

Magnesium: Even after being optimal on desiccated thyroid, I was shocked to find this too low, as was my potassium. Magnesium is a very important mineral, and when too low, can cause muscle cramping, heart palpitations, and constipation. When optimal, it supports your immune system and blood pressure, gives better energy.

Milk Thistle Seeds: This supplement has helped lower liver enzymes and high RT3. Recommended amounts start at 400 mg and research shows one can safely go up to 1200 mg daily. *We found it important to take iron supplementation with it, as milk thistle can slightly lower our serum iron.*

Minerals: Both in macro and trace, minerals are so important for health and well-being that thyroid patients put a strong emphasis on them. The macro-minerals include calcium, magnesium, potassium, sodium, phosphorus, chloride and sulfur and are needed in larger amounts by the body. Trace minerals iron, iodine, zinc, selenium, manganese, copper and cobalt are also important. Even fluoride is a trace mineral, but we get too much in our water.

Multivitamins: Opinions go back and forth as to the benefits of multivitamins. But on the positive side, they can do a great job filling in nutrient gaps if you don't eat certain foods. I prefer the raw whole food versions when I do use them.

Potassium: Like magnesium, many of us find ourselves low in the electrolyte potassium, which can cause salt retention and blood pressure problems. Potassium is important for good heart function, as well as skeletal and smooth muscle contraction, including for digestion. Long-term stress can also lower it. Requesting RBC (red blood cell) rather than serum will reveal cellular levels of potassium. Normal range can be 3.7 to 5.2, and research suggests healthy levels are mid-to-upper range. *Since too-high, over-the-range potassium can be dangerous, wise doctors recommend frequent lab testing.*

Powdered Greens: If you are like me and not big on veggies, this may be a good supplement to consider here or there. There are a variety of brands of powdered greens, and you will need to check the ingredients, as some have soy, which can be a no-no for thyroid patients. Many do not. It can be mixed with your morning liquid of choice, like juice or water with lemon juice. For that extra pizzazz, you can add flavored liquid stevia.

Probiotics: Having plenty of good bacteria is very important for our immune system, no matter if you have Hashimoto's or not. But it can be especially important to consider probiotics, the good bacteria in supplement form, if you do have Hashi's, to support and counter your haywire immune system. Multi-strain supplements are highly recommended.

Rhodiola Rosea (Golden Root): This plant helps alleviate depression, besides promote better energy and cognition. It's said to help the adrenals spread cortisol better throughout the day and counter stress, which is especially helpful if you have low cortisol! It's meant to support healthy adrenal function in the face of stress, too, or even out the highs and lows of cortisol.

Selenium: This has become a huge supplement for thyroid patients. The mineral selenium is not only potentially anti-cancer, it is part of the enzyme that causes T4 to convert to T3. Selenium is also a chelator of excess mercury, which we get from our fillings. Studies also find that selenium can lower Hashimoto's anti-TPO antibodies. The recommended safe maximum intake is 400 mcg.

Sea Salt: Salt is crucial for good adrenal function, and sea salt is the sodium of choice thanks to its trace minerals. Most patients will use ¼ to ½ tsp sea salt in a glass of water, especially in the morning and again in the late afternoon, in both stressful situations as well as with confirmed adrenal dysfunction or low aldosterone. *But if blood pressure is high, check with your doctor.*

Vitamin A: It seems that Vit. A is needed for thyroid hormones to absorb their needed iodine. And with hypothyroidism, your body has a reduced ability to convert beta carotene to Vit. A. So it's crucial for good immune function, besides vision and more. Ask a professional about amounts, since too much Vit. A is not good, either.

Vitamin C: Turns out that some thyroid patients who were on high-dose Vitamin C escaped the fall into adrenal dysfunction after being on T4 or being undiagnosed due to the lousy TSH lab test. The adrenals use more Vitamin C than another part of the body. Vit. C also makes the iron you take more absorbable, besides counters the free radicals caused by the iron. It also plays a role in thyroid hormone formation.

Vitamin D: Like B12 and ferritin/iron, many thyroid patients find themselves with low levels of this important vitamin, and it may explain the bone problems hypothyroid patients find themselves with. Vit. D is also mentioned as improving immune function as well as having a protective role against cancer and heart disease. When deficient as revealed by labs, we have found that most of us need to supplement with 10,000 IU's for a few weeks or less, then retest D3. We also take K2 with the D3 supplement to help move calcium to our bones.

Vitamin E: This is a fat-soluble vitamin with great benefits as an antioxidant against free radicals! Thus, it would be an excellent supplement if you ever are detoxing heavy metals. Plus, being hypothyroid is known to increase oxidative stress, so Vitamin E would be a good way to counter it until you can get out of the hypothyroid state.

Zinc: Besides improving one's immune system, zinc is needed for many enzymes to do their job, says the Linus Pauling Institute. So if labs reveal zinc is low, it can be good to supplement. But if you have low cortisol, zinc may need to be avoided since it has cortisol-lowering results. *Long-term zinc supplementation, such 50 mg daily, can lower copper levels.*

Everything listed in this chapter is not exhaustive, but just touches on some very important supplements and foods to consider. Want to test nutrients?
I love this one:

https://www.spectracell.com/patients/patient-micronutrient-testing/

GOOD FOODS, GOOD SUPPLEMENTS

* Potassium supplementation has helped many thyroid patients lower high blood pressure, but it's important to monitor your levels, since too-high potassium, i.e. over the range, can be dangerous.

* Research has shown that having low levels of selenium can promote too-high levels of Reverse T3.

* Zinc is known to lower cortisol, so you may need to avoid it while working on low cortisol, or just take low amounts of zinc.

* Taking supplemental progesterone? Research shows a strong correlation between progesterone and higher aldosterone levels—good news for those with low aldosterone.

INGREDIENTS FOR DESICCATED THYROID AND MORE THYROID PRODUCTS

T he thyroid powder used in the prescription desiccated thyroid products comes from porcine thyroids which have been *frozen, minced, dried and milled into a fine powder.* It is obtained from pigs that can be used for food for humans. It meets the USP (United States Pharmacopeia) microbial requirements for the absence of Salmonella and Escherichia coli. *Several batches are combined.* Testing is then done to make sure it meets the established specifications.

According to older literature about desiccated thyroid, when it's dried, it must have a limit loss of no more than 6% of weight. It also must meet inorganic testing and must yield not less than 90% or more than 110% of the labeled amounts of T4 and T3. The labeled amounts must be within 10% (plus or minus) of 38 mcg T4 and 9 mcg T3 for each grain of the labeled content of thyroid (60 or 65 mg according to the manufactured product). To read more detail, see the *1995 USP 23 NF 18, pp. 2684-2685 & 1997 USPDI-Volume III-17th Edition, p. IV/518.* There may be newer guidelines.

Non-prescription versions are usually stated to be grass-fed bovine, often from New Zealand or Argentina.

****

1) To make any NDT work as intended, patients need the right amount of iron and cortisol to prevent bad reactions, plus find their optimal dose, which always seems to put the free T3 towards the top of the range and the free T4 midrange.

2) The TSH lab test natura̶̶̶̶̶̶below range on this product with no bone loss or hear̶̶̶̶s as doctors wrongly scare monger.

3) Descriptions of the thyro̶̶̶̶ ̶̶̶̶̶̶̶̶ents in NDT only mention T4 and T3 (and the synthetic names), but they contain all five natural thyroid ingredients: T4, T3, T2, T1 and calcitonin.

4) Information below is based on when this book was updated. There can be new NDT products appear on the market: fillers can change, etc.

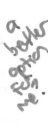

NP Thyroid: made by *Acella Pharmaceuticals, LLC.* This NDT first appeared in 2010, and patient reports on its use is highly positive. It can be done sublingually (under the tongue). The thyroid ingredients are listed as 38 mcg levothyroxine (T4) and 9 mcg liothyronine (T3) per one grain (60 mg), though like all desiccated thyroid, has all five hormones that aren't listed, but are there. Sometimes pharmacies will call it generic, but Acella says no, it's a name brand. So if you are substituted with NP Thyroid, it's a good thing. Ask the doc to put "NP Thyroid"by Acella" on the slip. Bad reviews are mostly based on patients not understanding to find their optimal amount (staying too low), or due to having inadequate iron or cortisol, which any NDT reveals. See *NPThyroid.com*

NP Thyroid has no wheat products in their tablets. Tablets are round, debossed on one side with "AP" and a 3-digit code on the other side as shown below:

> 15 mg (1/4 grain) – "327
> 30 mg (1/2 grain) – "329"
> 60 mg (1 grain) – "330"
> 90 mg (1 1/2 grain) – "331"
> 120 mg (2 grain) – "328"

Other ingredients include:
• Calcium Stearate
• Dextrose
• Mineral oil *(pharmaceutical grade and teeny tiny amount)*

Armour: made by Allergan/Activas, and still shows Forest Laboratories as a subsidiary. It is made in the following strengths: ¼, ½, 1, 2, 3, 4 and 5 grain tablets. The 3 and 5 grain tabs are scored. One grain is 60 mg and contains 38 mcg of T4 and 9 mcg of T3, plus unmeasured amounts of T2, T1 and calcitonin. The latter three are not removed, as rumor occasionally states. Each tablet contains (2018):
- porcine thyroid powder, U.S. Pharmacopeia
- calcium stearate (stabilizer and lubricant)
- dextrose
- microcrystalline cellulose
- sodium starch glycolate
- opadry white *(Titanium dioxide used as whitening agent, but may also contain trace amounts of PEG (polyethylene glycol), Polysorbate 80, and Hydroxypropyl Methylcellulose. Armour Thyroid is stated not to contain gluten or lactose.*
  http://www.armourthyroid.com
  https://www.allergan.com/assets/pdf/armourthyroid_pi

NatureThroid and WP Thyroid are distributed by RLC Labs, Inc. (formerly called Western Research Labs). Both are stated to be free of artificial colors, flavors, corn, peanut, rice, gluten, soy, yeast, egg, fish or shellfish. Naturethroid was first released in the 1930's!

Naturethroid ingredients are:
- *Porcine Thyroid Powder, U.S. Pharmacopeia (USP)*
- Colloidal Silicon *Dioxide (from mined ore: natural desiccant to protect from moisture and humidity)*
- Magnesium *Stearate (from a vegetable source like palm oil; lubricating agent for tablet compress)*
- Microcrystalline Cellulose *(synthetic fiber base to provide volume & bulk: also binds thyroid hormones, sadly)*
- Croscarmellose Sodium *(aids in disintegration in stomach and sadly, even more cellulose!)*
- Stearic *Acid (from vegetable source–typically palm oil; holds ingredients together)*
- Opadry II 85F19316 Clear – *tablet coating*

https://getrealthyroid.com/nature-throid.html
WP Thyroid comes in the following grain sizes: 1/4, 1/2, 3/4, one grain, 1 1/4, 1 1/2, Ingredients are:
- *Porcine Thyroid Powder, U.S. Pharmacopeia (USP)*
- Inulin derived from chicory root
- Medium chain triglycerides from coconut.

https://wpthyroid.com

History FYI: *Patients report that Naturethroid was reformulated in early 2010. The typical smell of desiccated thyroid was noted as less intense. The tablets were now stamped with RLC on one side, and N over 1 on the other, whereas before you'd see just NT1 or a reference to the fact that Time Caps Labs (TCL) used to make Naturethroid for RLC Labs. Calcium filler moved up from 16 mg to 17 mg/Potassium was removed. Cellulose seemed to become a problem.*

In 2017, patients saw both Naturethroid and WP Thyroid cease to be made--RLC stated updating the machinery. In 2018, Naturethroid first returned, and numerous patients reported a return of their symptoms, sooner or later. WP returned later that year and seemed to work again for most.

International:

Australia's Compounded thyroid: Porcine desiccated thyroid powder is imported to Australia and considered a food rather than a medicine. It's compounded by pharmacies and can be called thyroid extract. Patients report doing well with it and better than on T4. A patient asked Australian Custom Pharmaceuticals, Australia's largest compounding-only pharmacy, about their ingredients. It was stated that the only ingredients put in the capsules are the active ingredient (thyroid extract) and microcrystalline cellulose as the filler. At ACP 60mg (equivalent to 1 grain) contains 33.4 mcg T4 and 8.37 mcg of T3. However, together T4 and T3 may potentiate each other giving a therapeutic effect equivalent of 25 mcg of T3 and 100 mg of T4 per 60mg.

Canada's "Thyroid" by Erfa, formerly by Pfizer. They come in 30, 60 and 125 mg tablets and can be done sublingually the way Armour used to be. They contain:

- Dried Thyroid
- Magnesium Stearate
- Cornstarch
- Talc
- Sugar

History: Patients complained about Erfa's Thyroid not doing as well as it used to after May 2014.

Erfa's Canadian Thyroid has slightly different T4 and T3 ratios than the USP ratios of US brands.

In each Erfa 30 mg tablet embossed "ECI 30", there is 18 mcg of T4 and 4 mcg of T3 (as compared to 19/4.5 in US brands) This is equivalent to the US one-half grain.

In each Erfa 60 mg tablet embossed "ECI 60", there is 35 mcg of T4 and 8 mcg of T3 (as compared to 38/9 in US brands) This is equivalent to the US one grain.

In each Erfa 125 mg tablet embossed "ECI 125", there is 73 mcg of T4 and 17 mcg of T3 (as compared to 76/18 in US brands) This is equivalent to the US two grains.

http://eci2012.net/product/thyroid/

Denmark's Thyreoïdum from Biofac in Kastrup, Denmark. Imported into the Netherlands from BUFA/ Fargo, importers of pharmaceutical products.

½ grain = 29 mg (12.7 mg T4 and 4.5 mcg T3)

1 grain = 57 mg (25.3 mg T4 and 9 mcg T3)

2 grain = 114 mg (50.6 mg T4 and 18 mcg T3)

Pig thyroid. Some websites state the T4/T3 ratio can vary from 2.3: 1 to 3.8: 1 depending on the lot. Meets standards of US Pharmacopoeia. Contains Microcrystalline cellulose as a filler. Also may contain lactose, sodium, chloride, starch, sucrose or glucose.

https://natuurapotheek.com/index.php/en/news-and-information/thyreoidum-english

http://www.biofac.dk/products/thyroid-powder/

Germany's Thyreogland (SD Extrakt) from Munchen (Munich), Kloesterl Apoteke, Waltherstrasse, 80337 Muenchen. Phone: 089 *54343211 https://www.kloesterl-apotheke.de/* 1 grain Armour = 100 mcg levothyroxine = 40 mcg Thyreogland. Clear gelatin capsules with loose powder inside. May have magnesium stearate as a filler. The 25 mcg tablet specifies "25 mg T4 and circa 6 mcg T3_ on the label Also sent to me: the Kloesterl Apotheke (pharmacy) Munich Tel: 0049 (0)89 / 54 34 32 11 offers 4 different strengths: 25 mcgr T4+5.9 mcgr T3; 50 mcgr T4+11.8 mcgr T3; 75 mcgr T4+17.8 mcgr T3; 100 mcgr T4+23.7 mcgr T3. The 75 mcgr one is nearly exactly the equivalent of 2 grains of Armour. Also they add the amino acid tyrosine in the capsules as a filler. She advises all Germans to phone them and get the leaflet. It's more or less the only information about natural thyroid treatment available in Germany that one can take to a doctor.

Also available in Germany: compounded pork thyroid, aka Schilddruesen-Extrakt, in different grains

New Zealand's Whole Thyroid, which is compounded desiccated thyroid by Pharmaceutical Compounding New Zealand (PCNZ). Website: *http://www.pharmaceuticla.co.nz/*.

Non-prescription versions of NDT

Thyroid-S is from Sriprasit Pharma Co., Ltd. in Thailand (sister company of Sriprasit Dispensary R.O.P.) Advertising states that Sriprasit Pharma is "a leading importer of pharmaceutical products, and has been a GMP and ISO 9002-certified manufacturer of pharmaceutical products".

Patients report they are quite pleased with this product, but there are a lot of fillers. The ingredients, according to Pongsak Songpaisan of Sriprasit are:
- Thyroid extract USP
- Lactose (a milk sugar)
- PVP K90 (Polyvinylpyrolidone; water soluble coating;

- Avicel (microcrystalline cellulose; holds product together)
- Aerosil (silicic acid powder; help disperse the ingredients)
- Sodium starch glycolate (helps dissolute/disintegrate the pill)
- Magnesium stearate (filling agent)
- Eudragit (a common sustain released coating)
- Methocel (a water soluble cellulose ether-helps bind pill)
- Talcum (a filler)
- Ponceau 4r lake (red additive-aluminum)
- Tartrazine lake (yellow additive-aluminum)
- Brilliant blue FCF lake (blue additive-aluminum)
- Sunset yellow FCF (yellow additive)
- Titanium dioxide (white)
- PEG 6000 (water soluble polymer; binder)
- Dimethicone solution

In 2009, a US Doctor received the following list after emailing Sriprasit:

Fillers used: Corn starch, lactose, Avicel (microcrystalline cellulose; MCC) Binders used: PVP K-90 (Polyvinylpyrrolidone) Preservatives used: Methyl paraben, Propyl paraben Content in one tablet (60 mg thyroid extract): approximately 38 mg Levothyroxine (T4) and 9 mcg Liothyronine (T3) Source of extract: Porcine

Patient states: The Thyroid-S tablets are brown with a hard coating, they do not dissolve well as is, but can be chewed. They have a papaya like taste similar to "Thiroyd" below.

Thiroyd (yes, that's how they spell it) by Greater Pharma Ltd., a leading Thai Pharmaceutical Manufacturer. An email to a patient by Greater Pharma states that "thiroyd" at one grain contains T3 at 8.31 microgram; T4 at 35 mg, which is 0.013% and 0.058% respectively. A thyroid patient states: The Thiroyd tablets are white and have a sweet taste almost like papaya or a similar fruit. They dissolve very well sublingually and seem to have a very good potency. (Others say it does not dissolve well.) Entire paper insert with info is written in English: Greater Pharma Manufacturing Co. Ltd 55/2 Fillers may be lactose, tapioca Starch, sodium starch glycolate, PVP

K-30, PVP K-90, isopropyl alcohol, colloidal silicon dioxide, magnesium stearate.

Phutthamonthon, Nakhon, Pathom. Like Thyroid-S, this is ordered over the net.

ThyroGold is an over-the-counter dietary US desiccated thyroid product formulated by Dr. John C. Lowe and sold by his wife, Tammy. They contain freeze-dried bovine thyroid powder, 300 mg, from pasture-fed cows in New Zealand, as well as 25 mg Coleus forskohlii. Many patients like it.

There are many more versions of website-order natural desiccated thyroid on the net like Thyrovanz (*https://thyrovanz.com*) and others.

T3: Because there are so many brands of T3 and occasional changes, I keep T3 medications listed here: *http://stopthethyroidmadness.com/armour-vs-other-brands*
Knowing about T3 is important for those who have a reason to avoid porcine or bovine thyroid meds, and want to be on both T4 and T3, or have reason to be on T3 alone due to seriously high RT3 or a conversion problem.

T4: *If you do the two synthetics, Tirosint may be the best T4 to use with T3, as it's only got three other inactive ingredients: gelatin, glycerin, and water. Remember that even on both synthetics, we have to get optimal, not just be "on them".*

Ingredient Definitions:

Carnauba Wax - Derived from the pores of the leaves of the Brazilian wax palm tree. It is utilized in the final stage in tablet coating (to provide a complete seal).

Colloidal Silicon Dioxide - Derived from a mined ore. It is typically utilized as a natural desiccant in a tablet (to provide barrier from moisture and humidity).

Dicalcium Phosphate - Derived from a mined ore. It is typically utilized as a binder in a tablet (to hold all the ingredients during compression).

Hypromellose (Hydroxypropyl Methylcellulose) - Derived from a plant cellulose base (typically cotton blend and or wood pulp). It is typically utilized as a granulating agent in a tablet (to provide bulk and density to the tablet for proper compression) as well as part of a clear coating solution (with PEG).

Lactose Monohydrate - Derived typically from a dairy source. This ingredient is NOT added as a separate ingredient during formulation. It is a diluent base contributed from Thyroid USP powder (per USP monograph).

Magnesium Stearate - Derived from a vegetable source (typically palm oil). It is typically utilized as a lubricating agent in a tablet (to aid in proper compression of the tablet).

Microcrystalline Cellulose - Synthetically derived fiber (similar to plant-derived). It is typically utilized as a filler in a tablet (to provide volume and bulk).

Polyethylene Glycol (PEG) - Synthetically derived. It is utilized with Hydroxypropyl Methylcellulose as part of the clear coating solution.

Sodium Starch Glycolate - Synthetically derived starch molecule (similar to potato starch). It is typically utilized as a disintegrating agent in a tablet (to aid in proper disintegration of the tablet in the stomach).

Stearic Acid - Derived from a vegetable source (typically palm oil). It is typically utilized as a binder in a tablet (to hold all the ingredients during compression

VEGETARIAN, VEGAN, OR RELIGIOUS RESTRICTIONS ON THE USE OF PORK

There are two main reasons why someone might be concerned about the fact that prescription desiccated thyroid is from pigs: *vegetarianism, veganism, or religious practices.*

The practice of vegetarianism involves a strong belief in abstaining from the consumption of meat, fish, and poultry, which definitely includes pig, aka pork products. They may choose to eat dairy or eggs. Veganism also means abstaining from meat products, but might also include abstaining from other animal-derived products like egg and dairy. Either choice can be born from a variety of reasons: the quest for better health, religious beliefs, or political concerns about the treatment of animals.

Religious restrictions on the consumption of pork in specific are found in the Jewish and Muslim religions, as well as certain Christian Orthodox practices.

In these cases, the alternative to desiccated pig thyroid can be found in the use of adding Synthetic T3 to Synthetic T4, with the same goal of being optimal as on porcine or bovine desiccated thyroid, i.e a free T3 at the top part of the range, and a free T4 midrange. Both.

Your doctor can prescribe any of the above. Though some patients who take this route report that it didn't give them the excellent results that desiccated thyroid gives, it's the next best step from T4 alone and can work very well!

Another alternative is to consider the stance taken by Serene Shick. Serene is a vegan and Messianic. She found herself with many symptoms of hypothyroid, and did a great deal of research. She concluded that desiccated thyroid was her treatment of choice, in spite of her vegan choice:

All the evidence points to this being the superior medication for this illness, although most docs want to give the synthetics. NDT is all natural, which appeals to me in spite of the fact that it is derived from pigs. As you know, being vegan and Messianic, this doesn't sit well, but I have come to believe that what makes my body/brain/ temple perform optimally takes precedence over the desire to exclude all animal products from my diet as well as the mitzvah against pork. It is a very tiny amount and I am already feeling incredibly better: my thinking is clearer, I feel more in control of my emotions, and I am actually having frequent moments of real joy! So I am certain that YHVH has led me to this discovery.

As far as Judaism, the use of desiccated pig thyroid may be more tolerated if the tablet is swallowed rather than done sublingually, which may not violate Dietary Laws. Additionally, since the use of desiccated thyroid involves saving a life and mind, it may not be a problem.

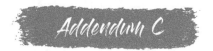

LABWORK DEFINITIONS PLUS HOW TO INTERPRET YOUR LABS

TSH:

Abbreviation for Thyroid Stimulating Hormone. Unfortunately, the TSH lab test has been the unfortunate darling of the medical establishment for potential diagnosis for thyroid disease. It's considered "a reliable gauge of your thyroid function as well as accurate guide to determine the right dose of thyroid medications" by medical professionals. It is not reliable at all. It's also considered a measurement of your own internal TSH which is secreted by your pituitary gland to stimulate your thyroid gland.

The standard normal range was 0.5 to 5.0, with hyperthyroid occurring below 0.5, and hypothyroid occurring above 5.0. In 2003, the American Association of Clinical Endocrinologists recommended that the new range be 0.3 to 3.04. To this day, some facilities still use the old range. Other ranges can be 0.4 to 4.5, or the highly ridiculous range from the UK of 0.5 to 10.0

Criticism: Patients have repeatedly found the TSH lab result to lag behind for years, even in the presence of obvious hypothyroidism and growing symptoms, before the result goes above the range to reveal hypothyroidism. Additionally, once on an optimal amount of desiccated thyroid, patients find their TSH lab result far below range, yet they have not one iota of hyperthyroid symptoms.

Benefits: The one area where the TSH is helpful is in the diagnosis of a pituitary dysfunction, especially Hypopituitarism.

If the TSH is low, in conjunction with a low free, and especially in the presence of hypothyroid symptoms, it's a clue that your pituitary is not functioning correctly.

Free T3:

Free represents what is unbound from protein and available for use and metabolically active. T3 (Triiodothyronine) is the active thyroid hormone. If not on medication, a high level would represent hyperthyroidism, and a low level would represent hypothyroidism.

On desiccated thyroid medication, the free T3 is at the upper end of the normal range. On T3-only, the free T3 is sometimes slightly over the top of the range, at the same time that all symptoms are removed (in the presence of strong adrenals or adequate cortisol, plus good blood pressure and heart rate). With low cortisol, the free T3 can be in the upper part of the range in the presence of continuing hypothyroid symptoms, called pooling, meaning it's not getting to the cells. It can also be low with a high Free T4, pointing to excess RT3.

Patients and certain doctors wisely recommend the use of this test for additional information.

Free T4:

Free represents what is unbound from protein and available for use. T4 (Thyroxine) is the storage thyroid hormone meant to convert to the active hormone T3, as needed. If not on medication, a high level would represent hyperthyroidism, and a low level would represent hypothyroidism.

On desiccated thyroid medication when optimal, many patients find their free T4 is approximately mid-range along with a free T3 at the top part of the range, at the same time that all symptoms are removed.

Patients and certain doctors wisely recommend the use of this test for additional information.

T3 (i.e. Total T3, not recommended by patients):

Without a *free* in front, this is the Total T3, or the total amount of both usable and non-usable   circulating thyroid hormone. It may be useful in the diagnosis of hyperthyroid, but patients and certain doctors find this test useless for hypothyroid diagnosis, since there is no idea what part of the result represents what is available for use. Additionally, pregnant women tend to naturally have higher total T3.

T4 (i.e. Total T4, not recommended by patients):

Without a *free* in front, this is the Total T4, or the total amount of both usable and non-usable   circulating thyroid storage hormone, which represents more the 99% of the T4. It may be useful in the diagnosis of hyperthyroid, but patients and certain doctors find this test useless for hypothyroid diagnosis, since there is no idea what part of the result represents what is available for use.

Reverse T3 (RT3):

A measure of the inactive form of T3. T4 converts to RT3 normally when the amount of T4 isn't needed, after surgery or an accident, or during an acute illness. But in the presence of high cortisol, low iron, low B12 and other chronic conditions, T4 can convert to excess amounts of RT3, which in turn, compete with the same cell receptors as T3. It's recommended that the RT3 lab test be done at the same time as a free T3 to compare the ratio. See Chapter 12.

Anti-TPO or Anti-thyroid Peroxidase Antibodies:

A measure of the antibodies which attack your thyroid peroxidase, an enzyme that plays a part in the production of thyroid hormones and T4 to T3. Helps diagnose Hashimoto's disease along with the TgAb lab test below. TPO antibodies can also be found with Graves' disease, though lower.

TgAb/Anti- Thyroglobulin Antibodies:

A measure of the antibodies which attack the key protein in the thyroid gland–the thyroglobulin–essential in the production of the T4 and T3 thyroid hormones. Along with the Anti-TPO, helps diagnose Hashimoto's disease.

Some patients find that they can be normal in one antibodies test and not in another, so *both TPO and TgAb are recommended to diagnose Hashimoto's disease.*

T3 Resin Uptake/T3RU (not recommended by patients):

A test that measures the level of thyroid hormone-binding proteins in the blood. Can be used to diagnose hyperthyroidism along with other tests.

Patients and certain doctors find this test unnecessary when hypothyroidism is suspected and is a general waste of your money.

Free Thyroxine Index (FTI or T7)
(not recommended by patients):

Along with the T4 and T3 Uptake, this test tells you how much thyroid hormone is free and unbound. It has been replaced by the free T4 test.

Patients and certain doctors find this test unnecessary when hypothyroidism is suspected and is a general waste of your money.

TRH:

Abbreviation for *TSH Releasing Hormone.* In your body, the TRH is released by the hypothalamus in order to tell the pituitary to release TSH. This test will see if the TSH goes up enough after the administration of the TRH. If your TSH goes up too far after the TRH is administered, it implies you may be hypothyroid. If you already have too much thyroid hormone, the administered TRH will not cause a rise in the TSH, making the test sensitive in detecting early hyperthyroidism.

This test is also used for cancer patients to see if they are on enough medication, or to ascertain the functioning of your pituitary gland.

This test is not used much anymore, since clinicians feel the TSH test alone replaces it.

TSI:

Abbreviation for Thyroid Stimulating Immunoglobins which will implicate Graves' hyperthyroid as well as Graves' ophthalmopathy or pretibial myxedema (bugged eyes). Rather than destroying tissue, the TSI antibodies react with your TSH receptors, causing them to tell your thyroid to produce far more. Some Hashimoto's patients can also have elevated TSI lab test.

Thyroid Scan or Radioactive Iodine Uptake:

This test is usually ordered by your doctor if there is an enlargement of your thyroid. It will produce a picture to help evaluate lumps or inflammation.

There are two types: one simply a scan to produce the picture, and the other is a *Radioactive Iodine Uptake*, which measures the absorption in your thyroid after you are given a dose of radioactive iodine in pill form. The amount of iodine detected in your thyroid will correspond to the amount of hormone your thyroid is producing.

Scans help identify whether nodules are hot or cold (determining possible cancer). Hot nodules are not usually cancerous.

Criticism: some patients have felt like the use of the scan was overkill when it was simply obvious they had Hashimoto's disease, which is treated with adequate doses of desiccated thyroid, and in many, the removal of gluten from their diet.

Ultrasound:

This is a test which uses sound waves in a high frequency to produce an image of your thyroid gland and possible nodules. It will tell your doctor if nodules found are solid or fluid filled and their size. It does not ascertain cancer. An ultrasound can also be helpful if someone has Seronegative Hashimoto's disease, a situation where neither of the normal antibodies are high.

Criticism: some patients have felt like the use of the ultrasound was overkill when it was simply obvious they had Hashimoto's disease, which is treated with optimal doses of desiccated thyroid or T4/T3, and in most, the removal of gluten from their diet plus any reactive foods.

Thyroid Needle Biopsy (thyroid FNA):

This test involves putting a very fine needle through your skin and into your thyroid to obtain a sample of your tissue, to tell whether a nodule is from cancer or is benign. It's thought to be safe, easy and an effective method to know whether you have cancer or not.

24-Hour Cortisol Saliva:

Those with healthy adrenal function will have the following results:

8 am: at the top of the range
11 am-noon: upper quarter, closer to the bottom part
4-5 pm: mid-range
bedtime: at the very bottom.

In the first stages of adrenal stress, you'll see higher and higher results. **In the next stages,** when the adrenals are falling over the hill, you'll see a mix of highs and lows. **In the more severe stages,** you'll see three or more lows, moderate or severe.

Alphabetical:

AB (Antithyroglobulin) Test for Hashimoto's: Generally, if this is above the range, you've got the autoimmune thyroid disease Hashi's. It the result is below the "less than" mark, or in the range provided, you may be fine, but you need to have done the other antibody test, TPO, as well. If either are below or "in" the range, but moving up, time to support your immune system. (See Chapter 8.)

ACTH Stim: Your cortisol levels will double if your adrenals are not diseased.

Aldosterone: An adrenal hormone which helps regulate levels of sodium and potassium in your body. If you are mid-or-below in the range, there is reason to be suspicious that your you have low aldosterone, since healthy levels will generally put you in the upper range.

This is best tested in the morning with no salt intake for 24 hours. Women need to do it in the first week after their period, since rising progesterone can also raise your aldosterone. Testing should not be done with severe illness (aldosterone falls in response to severe illness), during periods of intense stress (aldosterone rises), or right after strenuous exercise (aldosterone rises). Being pregnant can result in doubled amounts of aldosterone.

B12: We are looking for an optimal B12 lab result in the top quarter of the range, we have noticed repeatedly. It is not optimal to simply be "in range". If your range is similar to 180-900, a healthy level is approximately 750ish or higher. Methylcobalamin is a B12 supplement of choice, but others can work. It has been shown in studies that patients with labs under 350 are likely to have symptoms, which means the deficiency is very serious and has gone on for a few years undetected. It is suggested that lab ranges are much too low for B12; in Japan the bottom of the range is 500.

The urine test Urinary Methylmalonic Acid, also called the UMMA, can be added since it is a very sensitive detection and if high, will reveal a true B12 deficiency.

DHEA: as the mother of all steroid & sex hormones, DHEA is said to fall every decade, so supplementation can help in lower amounts.

Iron tests: There are four key iron tests:

> **Serum iron**
> **% saturation**
> **TIBC**
> **Ferritin**

Treating serum iron is the primary goal. It's not about ferritin alone as some doctors wrongly believe. We do get information from ferritin, such as inflammation. But for iron levels in general, it's about serum iron.

In US standard ranges and with no iron problem, **women** are close to 110 for serum iron, close to 35% for saturation, lower 300's or less for TIBC, and higher than 50 for ferritin, with a goal of 70-90. **Men** will have a serum iron in the 130's, % saturation around 38ish, TIBC in the lower 300's or less, Ferritin around 110ish. Those are the same goals when supplementing.

In Canadian and some European ranges that are less broad and go up to 30ish, serum iron for **women** is approximately 23ish, % saturation close to .35, TIBC lower 300's or less, ferritin 50's and higher. For **men**, optimal serum iron is towards the top of the range, % saturation around .38ish, TIBC lower 300's or less, ferritin 110's.

Ferritin can go too high due to inflammation, which has a variety of causes: antibodies attack from Hashimoto's, chronic infections, just being hypothyroid, any inflammatory diseases, and more.

Folate: Also called folic acid, this is a b-vitamin which can be low in hypothyroid patients. Folate is important for prenatal development, as well as your blood cell health and a treatment for the MTHFR mutation. Folate works with B12 in the use and creation of proteins.

Free T3: Those on an optimal amount of desiccated thyroid, with no lingering hypothyroid symptoms and in the presence of healthy adrenals, tend to have a free T3 at the top of the range. If it's lower, patients see their hypothyroid come back.

If the free T3 is high in the range with continued hypothyroid symptoms, that is called pooling, meaning T3 is not getting to the cells due to a cortisol problem, mostly low cortisol but can happen with high.

If not on thyroid medication: 1) If your free T3 (and free T4) is high, you could have Hashimoto's disease, which will need the two antibodies tests to discern it, or Graves' disease, which needs the TSI test. 2) If your free T3 is mid-range or lower, and in the presence of hypothyroid symptoms, you may have hypothyroidism, no matter how low the TSH. 3) If your free T3 is low and free T4 is high, you need to look at your RT3 (Chapter 12)

Free T4: Those on an optimal amount of desiccated thyroid will generally find this mid-range along with a free T3 at the top, and in the presence of healthy adrenal function. Those on T3-only will find their free T4 very low.

Magnesium (RBC, aka Red Blood Cell rather than Serum): You are looking for an RBC magnesium result mid-range or slightly higher.

Potassium (RBC, aka Red Blood Cell rather the Serum): Generally, a healthy potassium level is in the upper part of the range. If too high, it's called hyperkalemia; when too low, hypokalemia. It can rise in the presence of low aldosterone, then fall.

Renin: Done in conjunction with the aldosterone tests. If renin is high in the range along with a low aldosterone, you have an adrenal cause. If both hormones are low in the range, you could have a pituitary problem. Always tested along with Aldosterone to see if your problem is due to the adrenals (primary adrenal insufficiency) or your pituitary (secondary adrenal insufficiency).

Reverse T3 (RT3): This test has to be done at the same time you do the free T3. Healthy levels put the RT3 in the bottom two numbers of any range, or 3rd from the bottom at the most. (Chapter 12.)

Sodium: Healthy levels are midrange and higher. Or if a range is 135-145, healthy levels seem to be around 142.

Thyroid Peroxidase Antibody (TPO) test for Hashimoto's: Generally, if this is above the range, you've got the autoimmune thyroid disease Hashimoto's. If the result is below the "less than" mark, or in the range provided, you may be fine, but you need to do the other antibody test. (Chapter 8.)

TIBC (Total iron binding capacity) test: measures whether a protein called transferrin, produced by the liver, has the ability to carry iron in the blood. Used to determine anemia or low body iron. It your result is high, and in the absence of chronic disease, you can be anemic.

TSH: Creators of the TSH lab test came up with a range that supposedly corresponds with healthy thyroid function. So theoretically, if your TSH lab results are higher than the range, it would imply something is triggering your actual TSH to be a little too active in screaming at your thyroid. That something would be a diseased thyroid, called hypothyroid, or any reason to be hypothyroid.

But there are problems with this method of diagnosis. First, you can have a so-called normal result, yet be clearly hypothyroid with symptoms. Why? Because the TSH test cannot measure if all your cells & tissue are receiving the released thyroid hormones. Some may be (thus the normal TSH result) and some may not be (thus your clear symptoms). Second, if you have Hashimoto's, your lab results can swing between hypo- and hyper, & your lab test may be representing the middle of the swing.

The best way to use the TSH lab test is in diagnosing a pituitary problem, not a thyroid problem. When not on meds, a very low TSH with a low free T3 gives away a pituitary issue.

Vitamin D: (25-hydroxyvitamin D):   50-80 at the minimum is your goal in the range: 80-100 is considered cancer protective, say some experts. Many thyroid patients are low in D due to digestive issues from being undiagnosed or undertreated, plus problems with Celiac or gluten intolerance.

T7, Total T3, Total T4, Uptake, or any other thyroid labs: A waste of your money and blood, exclaim thyroid patients.

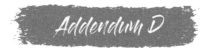
LABS, LAB FACILITIES, AND PREPARATION

L abs are important. They give us key information that just going by symptoms may not!

For example, and with thyroid labs in particular like the **Free T3** and **Free T4,** they are quite critical. Why? Because on NDT, or T4/T3 or even T3-only, we have made a mistake by stopping at the amount of meds that made us "feel good" without checking those labs. Thus, the "feeling good" backfired on us eventually, and our symptoms returned.

So if feeling good is not a clue as to our right amount, what is? It's those lab results! We have to be "optimal" in those ranges with our Free T4 and Free T3. Optimal has for years with patients put the Free T3 at the top part of the range and the Free T4 midrange. Both. And when they are optimal, our feel-goods last! We don't see a return of our hypothyroid symptoms as we do if we just stop at "feeling good".

Jeanne is an example:

I got on desiccated thyroid and after two raises and up to 2 grains, I felt remarkable. So I stayed there, happy, more active. I'm a 68 year old grandma so this was a miracle. But after about 3 months, it all went down the drain. I was sleepy in the afternoons again, and I felt wired, weepy, and very defensive with my husband. I headed back to the book and suspected I now had an adrenal problem. I ordered a saliva cortisol test and there it was. My morning and noon were low and the other two were high. So 2 grains was always underdosing me. I knew about the optimal goals. I should have done labs. I had to get on adrenal cortex to treat the lows, and I took holy basil to treat the highs. Today, I'm not optimal at 3 ¼ grains. My Frees are exactly where Janie says they are for people over the years who both feel good and don't see it reverse.

With other labs, being non-optimal may not be as obvious... at first. Examples are **B12, Vitamin D, other vitamins, and minerals.** But the problems from not being optimal are destined to show themselves eventually. i.e. what causes non-optimal levels can still be going on, pushing levels further down. Again, it underscores how important lab work is to help us find our optimal sweet spot.

We also need all **four iron labs, both thyroid antibodies.**

Speaking of doing lab work, no more are some patients held hostage to having to pay to visit a doctor and get a prescription for labs. If you can afford it, there are a growing amount of self-order lab facilities. Even a saliva cortisol test can be sent to you in legal areas. Then, if you so desire, you can share the results with your doctor at a future visit.

Below are a few examples of self-test facilities where you can order your own labs. You then print out the form and take it to most any draw location. The US listed facilities have affiliated links, meaning that if you order via the link, the facilities provides a small percentage to help with the hosting cost of the huge Stop the Thyroid Madness website.

1. United States

ULTA LAB TESTING (in the US):

This has been a very popular facility to order one's own lab work. To get 10% off, use this ULTA41012. If you find the latter has expired at any point in time you are reading this book, just email them and ask for new one. *https://www.ultalabtests. com/sttm/Shop/Promotion/6262*

DIRECT LABS (in the US):

This is a friendly facility and even has a heavy metal hair test. *https://www.directlabs.com/sttm/OrderTests.aspx*

MY MED LAB (in the US) (has a great saliva cortisol test!):
An excellent saliva test: *http://tinyurl.com/saliva-cortisol*
This self-ordering lab facility has lab packages designed
specifically for readers of Stop the Thyroid Madness, including
one of the best saliva tests out there.

2. Canada
Patients can order from these: *https://bloodtestscanada.
com/, https://www.truehealthlabs.com/category-s/1975.htm*

**For other countries: Because self-ordering facilities
are appearing all the time, I suggest going to the internet and
doing a search for self-ordering lab facilities.

Labs and Preparation

• **Thyroid:** We have learned repeatedly NOT to take our
thyroid meds before we test. We just take our thyroid meds as
usual the day before the lab test (though we bring any evening
thyroid meds to the daytime), and do testing the next morning
before taking thyroid meds for that day. We always want to see
what we are holding into. *Optimal: free T3 towards the top
part of the range, and the free T4 midrange*
• **Saliva cortisol:** Saliva is critical, not blood, as blood
is mostly measuring bound cortisol. Saliva measures what
is available. And because we want to test what is going on
naturally with our cortisol levels, and not what is influenced,
we attempt to be off any adrenal support or herbs for 1-2 weeks
before doing saliva testing, *if possible.*
*Optimal: morning at the tip top of the range; Noonish in the
upper quarter, but nearer the bottom part of upper quarter; Late
afternoon should be midrange; Bedtime at the very bottom.*
• **Aldosterone:** We have learned to be totally off salt for a
minimum of 24 hours before our test, since sodium can affect
the test. We want to see what is going on without influence. We
move around for the day at least an hour before testing, and we
test in an upright position, not laying down. For women: Since

progesterone needs to be at its lowest, we test anywhere from the start of the menstrual flow until a week afterwards. Close to 8 am is ideal when aldosterone levels are at the highest. Testing sodium and potassium at the same time is ideal, since low aldosterone could affect these minerals. *Optimal aldosterone: much above midrange.*

• **Electrolytes (Potassium and Sodium, which can be negatively affected by low aldosterone):** Some recommendations state to avoid these minerals the day before; others say to simply fast and avoid them on the day of the test until after your test is done. *For sodium and in a range of 135-145, it should be 140-142, we have noted. Potassium should not be low in the range. For potassium testing, remind the lab tech to avoid using the tourniquet, since prolonged use can give a false high reading of potassium.*

• **B12:** We stop eating or drinking the night before. i.e. fasting for the blood draw. *Optimal: upper quarter of range is where we see all symptoms gone of low B12.*

• **Iron testing:** If not on any iron supplements, we can test right away the next morning after fasting. If we are taking any iron supplements or eating iron rich foods, we stay off for up to 5 days before testing, in order to see what we are holding onto. *Optimal serum iron for women is ~110 for women, ~130's for men. If ferritin is above the 90's for women, or above 110's for men, it points to inflammation, which we'd have to treat before being on iron...otherwise, iron is thrust into storage ferritin.*

• **Vitamin D:** Fasting the night before the morning test is ideal. *Optimal: for the 25-hydroxyvitamin D blood test, we prefer to ourselves in the 40-60 range minimum.*

• **Sex hormones:** We found this more accurate with blood testing, not saliva. If we are already supplementing with hormones, we do testing 12 hours after our last dose, i.e. taking none before the lab draw.

• **Copper and zinc:** We have seen so many with a copper/zinc imbalance that this is worthy mention. i.e. when testing both, you want up to 8 times more zinc than copper. Another way to look at it is that you want your ratio between the two to be should be .7 – 1.0. Also test RBC zinc.

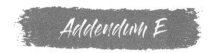

HOW To FIND
A GOOD DoCToR

A needle in the haystack can best describe how hard it is for patients to find a good doctor for knowledgeable thyroid and adrenal care. There is hardly a patient alive who hasn't encountered doctors who make some or all of the following mistakes, even to this day:

- Ordering lab tests that are lousy in detecting hypothyroidism, such as the TSH and total T4
- Holding you hostage to the TSH lab test, which keeps you underdosed
- Viewing lab ranges as from God Almighty
- Prescribing only T4-only medications
- Being completely ignorant about the efficacy of desiccated thyroid, or even T3
- Telling you that you need to exercise more and eat less
- Having poor knowledge about our cortisol issues and how to treat them
- Dismissing your own wisdom about the body you live in
- Putting you on other medications which end up bandaiding a poor thyroid treatment
- Sending you to other doctors as if the answer to your continued problems is mysterious or in need of a "specialist" like an Endocrinologist

But if you work hard and do your homework, you may succeed in finding one who will do most of it, if not all, correctly, as outlined in Chapter 3: What Thyroid Patients Have Learned: the Bible of our Experience. *Or, at the very least,* you can find a doctor who is open-mined to what you have learned from this book and the experiences of hundreds of thousands of thyroid patients. i.e. you find on you can teach!!

So conversely to the first list of mistakes that doctors make, a good doctor is one who knows, or can be taught that....

- Desiccated thyroid or T3 has always worked better than simply T4.
- It's about the Free T3 and Free T4 and being "optimal", not just anywhere in the range.
- Optimal has always put our Free T3 at the top part of the range and Free T4 midrange. Both.
- If we have problems raising NDT or T3 with bad symptoms, that points to a cortisol or iron problem.
- Saliva cortisol is the best way to test our cortisol levels, not blood.
- Iron testing is not about just testing ferritin. It's about serum iron, % saturation, TIBC and ferritin.
- To rule out autoimmune Hashimoto's, both antibodies labs are needed, not just one.
- It is not about holding us hostage to the TSH.
- It is natural for the TSH to go below range on NDT or T3 and as one is approaching optimal.
- We will not get bone loss or heart disease from our suppressed TSH on NDT or T3.

So how do you find a good doc who is either knowledgeable or who can be taught by you?

1. **Ask a Pharmacist:** A successful way to find a potentially 'better' doctor is to approach/call the Pharmacist, and ask for names of doctors they have seen who prescribe desiccated thyroid or T3. Most Pharmacists or their techs are usually friendly and will let you know. Don't hesitate to call or go to more than one pharmacy.

2. **Check out good Physician Groups websites:** Try the American College for the Advancement for Medicine website at *www.acam.org/*, or the Functional Medicine website at *www.functionalmedicine.org/*, or doctors

who are board certified in Environmental Medicine here: *www.aaemonline.org/*.

3. **Find a Functional Medicine doctor or an Osteopath (DO):** Though no doctor is perfect, you are more likely to find better doctors about thyroid treatment in those specialties.

4. **Saliva Lab Facility listing of doctors:** A doctor who uses saliva labs may be a doc more open-minded about desiccated thyroid, and perhaps even cortisol.

5. **Patient feedback/word of mouth:** Check out this page for groups: *http://stopthethyroidmadness.com/ talk-to-others*

6. **Older doctors:** Some of the oldest doctors who are still practicing are likely to remember the successful use of desiccated thyroid and may be open to using it.

7. **Patient groups:** Yes, some thyroid social media groups keep a list of better doctors in their Files.

BEWARE: Just because a doctor advertises him or herself as a thyroid doctor has not mean they are caught up with our knowledge!

IMPORTANT TO REMEMBER: *No doctor is going to be perfect. They are busy; some are extremely closeminded. And poor medical school training, rigid licensing boards, brainwashing pharmaceutical reps, and their continuing education makes them imperfect.*

So no matter how wonderful a doc looks, you have to be your own best advocate by being knowledgeable when you walk in. Be friendly yet firm about what is right for you. Stop giving your power away when you enter the doctor's office. It's your body and intelligence from reading this book, and your wisdom, too.

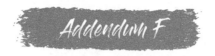
INTERPRETING YOUR CORTISOL SALIVA LAB RESULTS

The following information was brilliantly created and compiled by Bob Harvey, a thyroid, adrenal and hypopituitary patient. It is based on the DiagnosTechs saliva test, *but you do not have to use their saliva test to benefit from this information.* Another good one is this: *https://tinyurl.com/saliva-cortisol* He also uses some information from Genova Labs and ZRT. It is his hope that you will gain better understanding about your saliva cortisol lab work and the stages of your adrenal dysfunction as you work closely with your doctor.

* * * * *

The first lab to test cortisol levels in the saliva was DiagnosTechs. Their web site has a list of doctors that use the lab, and if you have trouble finding a Doctor near you, the lab kit can be ordered directly by the patient 3.

Unlike a single blood draw in the morning, the DiagnosTechs lab result shows the amount of cortisol at 4 points of the day. The main things you are looking for in your cortisol labs are:

1. The quantity of cortisol, high or low.
2. The rhythm. You want it to be as normal as possible.

In the first figure the cortisol is a bit higher than normal. Doctor Hans Selye theorized that elevated cortisol is the body's initial reaction to stress.

The solid black line shows that this person's cortisol is higher than normal at the beginning and end of the day. The lab will print out the cortisol amounts from the 4 points in the day, compared to the normal range.

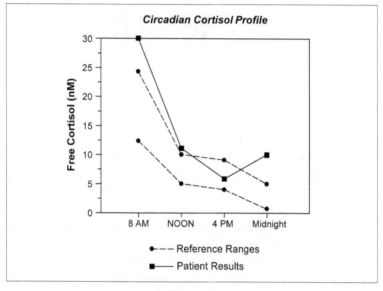

Figure-1.

Free Cortisol Rhythm			
07:00 - 08:00 AM	31	Elevated	13-24 nM
11:00 - Noon	11	Elevated	5-10 nM
04:00 - 05:00 PM	5	Normal	3-8 nM
11:00 - Midnight	9	Elevated	1-4 nM
Cortisol Burden:	56		23-42

Figure-2.

Do you see the term "cortisol burden"? (*See* Figure -2). This is the combined amounts of all 4 of the cortisol samples taken through the day. This person's value of "56" is higher than the normal range (23 - 42). This does not necessarily mean that this person will have lots of energy–many people with high cortisol describe symptoms of fatigue, anxiety, and insomnia (similar to low cortisol symptoms). High cortisol can impair the conversion of T4 (the "storage form" of thyroid hormone) into T3 (the "active form" of thyroid hormone).

DiagnosTechs labs have a grid showing numbers 1 - 7. This person's result is in the "normal" zone despite the high cortisol in the morning and night because this grid takes the readings from the noon and afternoon points of the day, and averages them to get a single value to put on this chart.

Do you see how the average of the noon and 4 pm cortisol amounts would place the black square in the "normal zone" above? It is a bit higher than normal, but still fits within the range.

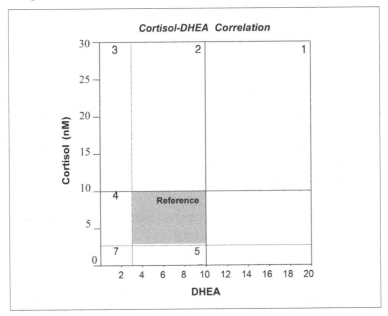

Figure-3.

That is the most "stable" part of the day in terms of the cortisol rhythm, and that is also when they gather the DHEA reading. The lab's explanation below says the correlation of cortisol to DHEA was in the (normal) reference zone, but there could still be high or low cortisol at specific points in the day.

Looking at the big picture, this person has high cortisol, and the rhythm is not normal.

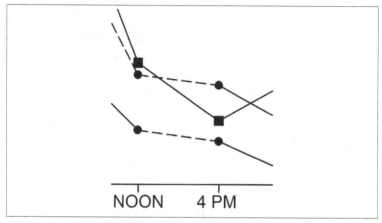

NOON   4 PM

Figure -4.

DHEA   Dehydroepiandrosterone
        Pooled Value   4   Normal   Adults (M/F): 3-10 ng/ml

Figure 3 shows your cortisol-DHEA correlation was in: Reference zone individuals in this zone usually display a balance in the average values of cortisol to DHEA for the day.

Falling in the reference zone does not preclude the occurrence of high or low cortisol at any specific time on their circadian.

Figure -5.

OK, let's look at another example where the person has high cortisol on the next page.

The combined cortisol throughout the day is 87, compared to a normal range of (23 - 42). This person's cortisol is DOUBLE the highest range of normal.

This person's DHEA is a bit higher than center of normal,

and if you look at the grid below, you will see that the black square is to the right of center, but still within the normal zone.

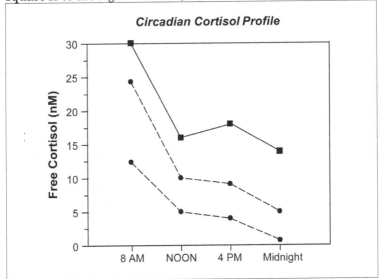

Figure -6.

Free Cortisol Rhythm			
07:00 - 08:00 AM	39	Elevated	13-24 nM
11:00 - Noon	16	Elevated	5-10 nM
04:00 - 05:00 PM	18	Elevated	3-8 nM
11:00 - Midnight	14	Elevated	1-4 nM
Cortisol Burden:	87		23-42
DHEA Dehydroepiandrosterone	8	Normal	Adults (M/F): 3-10

Figure -7.

On the next page, if you were to average the noon and 4 pm cortisol amounts, you can see how the black square ends up higher than normal.

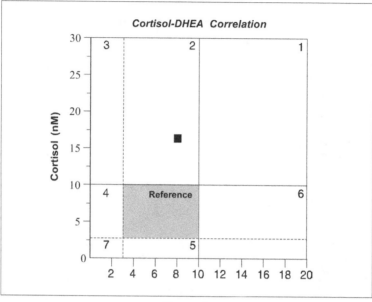

Figure -8.

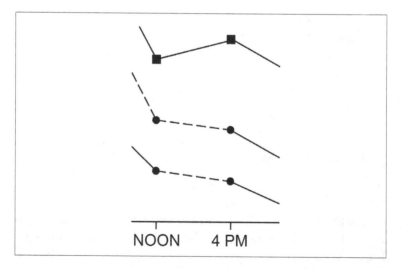

Figure -9.

DiagnosTechs has determined that the Cortisol to DHEA correlation is "Zone 2", that is where the black square is placed. If you look at the explanation below, this means "Adapted with DHEA slump". What does this mean?

If this person's DHEA lab result was higher, the little black square would be in "Zone 1". The explanation for Zone 1 "adapted to stress" means that the body is responding to the challenge. Healthy adrenals react to stress by putting out more cortisol, and the DHEA levels will increase in a similar way. In the example above, "Adapted with DHEA slump", the person's cortisol has adapted to the stress but the DHEA is not maintaining the higher output. If the DHEA was below normal, the black square would be in Zone 3.

The theory of the adrenals reaction to stress is explained on a web site by Dr. Lam beginning with the "Alarm" phase–increased cortisol as a reaction to stress.

During times of stress, the body requires more cortisol, and if this demand continues, more of the Pregnenolone will go toward cortisol–and less DHEA will be made.

KEY: CORTISOL-DHEA CORRELATION
1. Adapted to stress.
2. Adapted with DHEA slump.
3. Maladapted Phase I.
4. Maladapted Phase II.
5. Non-adapted, Low Reserves.
6. High DHEA.
7. Adrenal Fatigue.

Figure -10.

Now, please look at the DiagnosTechs grid of "7 Zones" once more. Can you visualize how the person is making plenty of DHEA at 1–then drops down at 2 and 3? The person still has high cortisol, but the DHEA levels are dropping.

As the adrenal fatigue progresses, Dr. Lam's site refers to the "Resistance" phase. He says "While the morning, noon, or afternoon cortisol levels are often low, the nighttime cortisol level is usually normal." This DiagnosTechs lab is an example where the morning cortisol has dropped down.

We really don't know if this person's adrenal fatigue was caused by stress, but it would fit Dr. Lam's explanation "With chronic or severe stress, the adrenals eventually are unable to keep up with the body's demand for cortisol. As such, the cortisol output will start to decline from a high back to a normal level, while the ACTH remains high. With protracted ACTH and adrenal fatigue, less cortisol is produced due to the adrenals becoming exhausted."

ACTH is an abbreviation for Adrenocorticotropic hormone, produced by the pituitary gland, which stimulates the adrenal glands to produce cortisol. An early morning blood test for the

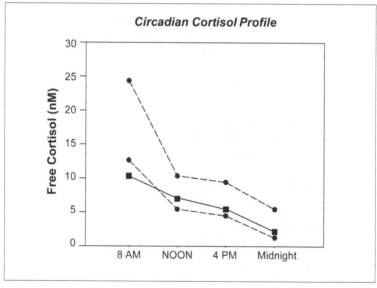

Figure -11.

ACTH levels would provide a more complete picture for this person. If the ACTH is high, yet cortisol is low, the problem is with the adrenals. But if the lab revealed low ACTH, the person could have some degree of hypopituitary.

As you read the complete Dr. Lam article, he explains that in this phase of adrenal fatigue the DHEA levels continue to drop, and this person would be an example of that. The lab result of "2" falls out of the normal DHEA range (3 - 10). Do you see how that has placed the little black square over to the left side of normal?

Free Cortisol Rhythm			
07:00 - 08:00 AM	10	Depressed	13-24 nM
11:00 - Noon	7	Normal	5-10 nM
04:00 - 05:00 PM	4	Normal	3-8 nM
11:00 - Midnight	2	Normal	1-4 nM
Cortisol Burden:	23		23-42
DHEA Dehydroepiandrosterone	2	Depressed DHEA	Adults (M/F): 3-10

Figure -12.

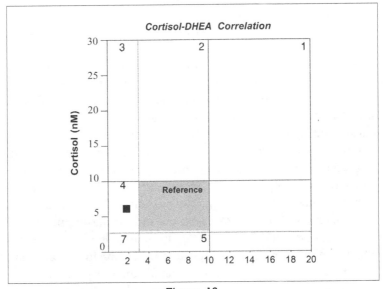

Figure -13.

As the person's DHEA gets lower, the black square moves

to the left.

Why is this person's cortisol in the normal range? Remember, DiagnosTechs uses the average of the mid-day readings to determine where the black square will go.

This lab happens to be from a relative who had symptoms of adrenal fatigue, especially waking up tired, craving coffee and sweets, and feeling best only after 6 pm[23].

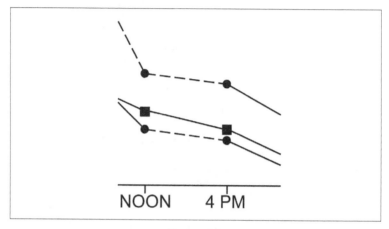

Figure -14.

At first glance, his labs don't look that bad. His cortisol burden is 23 compared to range (23 - 42). But the symptoms are important in deciding what to do. And remember what Dr. Lam says: "adrenal hormones are low in the case of adrenal fatigue, but still within the "normal" range and not low enough to warrant the diagnosis of Addison's disease by regular blood tests. In fact, your adrenal hormones can be half of the optimum level and still be labeled "normal". Such "normal" level of adrenal hormones does not mean that the patient is free from adrenal fatigue. Conventional doctors are not taught the significance of sub-clinical adrenal fatigue. They are misguided by blood tests which are not sensitive enough to detect sub-clinical adrenal. As a result, patients tested for adrenal functions are told they are "normal" but in reality, their adrenal glands are performing sub-optimally, with clear signs and symptoms as the body cries

---

[23] http://adrenalfatigue.org/doi.php

out for help and attention.

"Adrenal fatigue afflicts more people than Addison's disease. It is not recognized and has become an epidemic of massive proportion."

My relative evaluated his symptoms and the fact that he also had very low thyroid hormones. He did not want to begin thyroid supplementation without supporting the adrenals first.

He followed a good dosing protocol for Hydrocortisone (Cortef). He noticed improvement right away and is doing well. He was able to introduce a prescription for desiccated thyroid and did even better, with his temperatures finally coming up to normal.

* * *

Here's an example with less cortisol:

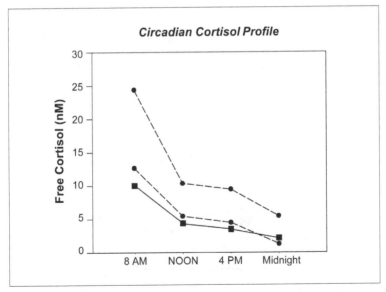

Figure -15.

DiagnosTechs will focus on the average of the Noon and 4 pm readings to determine where the black square goes. The DHEA is within normal range. This person is on the edge of zone 5, but the lab does consider it a zone 5 as explained below.

I think most of us could agree that this person has a low cortisol output. The cortisol burden (combined values) is 18 (23 - 42 normal range). The lab mentions that this condition is usually the outcome of stress—but really there is no way to say exactly what caused this person's condition without doing additional lab tests.

Free Cortisol Rhythm			
07:00 - 08:00 AM	10	Depressed	13-24 nM
11:00 - Noon	4	Depressed	5-10 nM
04:00 - 05:00 PM	2	Depressed	3-8 nM
11:00 - Midnight	2	Normal	1-4 nM
Cortisol Burden:	18		23-42

Figure -16.

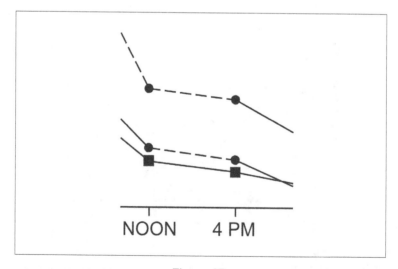

Figure -17.

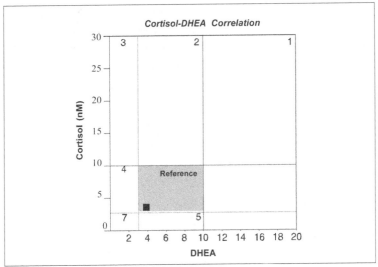

Figure -18.

DHEA   Dehydroepiandrosterone
Pooled Value   4   Normal Adults (M/F): 3-10 ng/ml

Figure 3 shows your cortisol-DHEA correlation was in: Zone 5 - Non-adapted, Low Reserves
This zone represents a suboptimal cortisol output reflecting an adrenal decline or a depleted reserve. The reduced demand for pregnenolone precursor in the cortisol pathway may allow a normal DHEA production. This condition is usually the outcome of chronic and protracted exposure to stressors.

Figure -19.

Here's an example with even less cortisol:
This person had immeasurable cortisol three of the points in the day, with a total combined cortisol burden of only 8 (range 23 - 42).
The average of the Noon and 4 pm readings would put the black square as low as it could go, because both readings were immeasurable. But because the DHEA was within the normal range, the black square goes to zone 5.

Do you see the explanation for Zone 5–"Non-adapted, Low Reserves"? They are assuming this person was subjected to stress. If they had "adapted" to the stress, they would be putting out high levels of cortisol. The cortisol is low, so they are "Non-adapted".

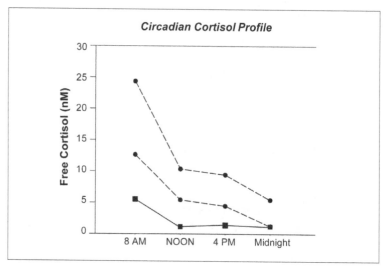

Figure -20.

Free Cortisol Rhythm			
07:00 - 08:00 AM	5	Depressed	13-24 nM
11:00 - Noon	<1	Depressed	5-10 nM
04:00 - 05:00 PM	<1	Depressed	3-8 nM
11:00 - Midnight	<1	Depressed	1-4 nM
Cortisol Burden:	8		23-42
DHEA Dehydroepiandrosterone	4	Normal	Adults (M/F): 3-10

Figure -21.

The "low reserves" means that if the person gets sick, or other increased stress, they lack the "reserves" to put out the increased cortisol that the body requires. Dr. Jefferies talks about this in his book *Safe uses of Cortisol.*

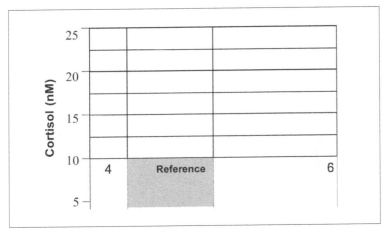

Figure -22.

KEY: CORTIAOL-DHEA CORRELATION
1. **Adapted to stress.**
2. **Adapted with DHEA slump.**
3. **Maladapted Phase I.**
4. **Maladapted Phase II.**
5. **Non-adapted, Low Reserves.**
6. **High DHEA.**
7. **Adrenal Fatigue.**

Figure -23.

You might think that a Zone 6 is worse than a Zone 5, but not necessarily.

This person has almost a perfect centerline normal "cortisol burden" of 30 (23 - 42) but the DHEA is way higher than normal.

Here you can see how the DHEA has shoved the black square far over to the right, and if the cortisol amounts from the average of Noon and 4 pm fall within the normal range, it is a Zone 6.

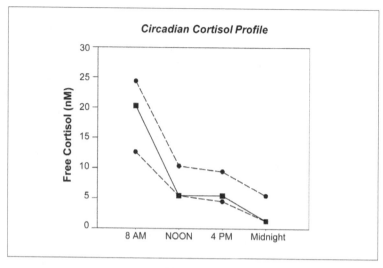

Figure -24.

Free Cortisol Rhythm			
07:00 - 08:00 AM	20	Normal	13-24 nM
11:00 - Noon	5	Normal	5-10 nM
04:00 - 05:00 PM	4	Normal	3-8 nM
11:00 - Midnight	1	Normal	1-4 nM
Cortisol Burden:	30		23-42
DHEA Dehydroepiandrosterone	19	Elevated DHEA	Adults (M/F): 3-10

Figure -25

There are examples of labs with the black square in Zone 6 that had lower cortisol, and I have seen some with cortisol so low that it lands in the area "below 6" that has no Zone number.

High DHEA is a problem. Dr. Peatfield says "High levels of cortisol and DHEA show adrenals under stress. Sometimes the cortisol pathway starts to fade as exhaustion sets in, with DHEA still reasonably present. Less commonly, there may be a really high DHEA–a response to ACTH stimulation but with the cortisol pathways responding poorly. Erratic levels in both are evidence of strain and uneven response."

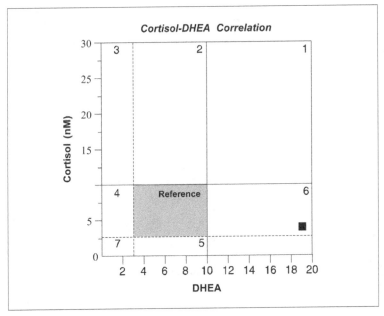

Figure -26.

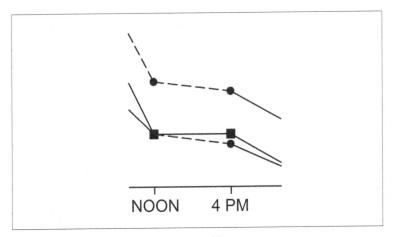

Figure -27.

Let's look at another example This person has low cortisol, especially in the mid-day, when DiagnosTechs focuses on where to put the little black square.

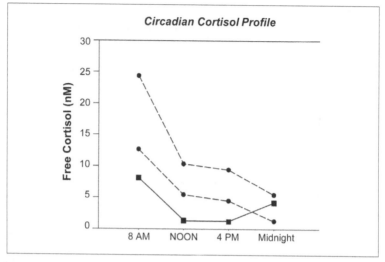

Figure -28.

Free Cortisol Rhythm			
07:00 - 08:00 AM	8	Depressed	13-24 nM
11:00 - Noon	1	Depressed	5-10 nM
04:00 - 05:00 PM	1	Depressed	3-8 nM
11:00 - Midnight	3	Normal	1-4 nM
Cortisol Burden:	13		23-42

Figure -29.

Because the DHEA was below normal, the black square ends up in Zone 7.

OK, so the lab is explaining low Cortisol and low DHEA. They say that taking steroids could cause a lab result like this and the instructions that come with the DiagnosTechs kit warn that the use of Hydrocortisone, Adrenal Cortex, etc. will affect the results. That is why you want to do these tests BEFORE treatment.

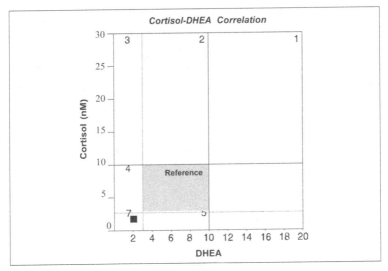

Figure -30.

DHEA
Pooled Value 2 Depressed DHEA Adults (M/F): 3-10 ng/ml

Figure 3 shows your cortisol-DHEA correlation was in: Zone 7 - Adrenal Fatigue
This zone represents a fatigue or suppression of the adrenals with overt deficits in either or both cortisol and DHEA production. Individuals with suppressed hypothalamic pituitary axis due to exogenous steroid overuse may also show results that fall in zone 7.

Figure -31.

This person had very low DHEA. People with hypo-pituitary often have low DHEA on lab tests, so it isn't always a simple matter of "stress" or fatigued adrenals.

* * *

Let's look at another "Zone 7" example. Zone 7's is not always "flat-lining".

Because of the high morning cortisol, this person's total cortisol output for the day "28" is within the normal range (23 - 42). But the DHEA is below normal.

Why did the black square end up in "Zone 7"? Remember, DiagnosTechs uses the midday average to place the little black square.

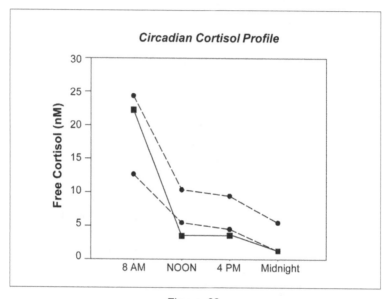

Figure -32.

* * *

This person has the low morning cortisol, with normal levels later in the day, which indicates adrenal fatigue.

The average of the Noon and 4 pm cortisol levels fit within the normal range. The DHEA fit within the normal range, so this person's "Zone" is normal. But the cortisol burden of 19 falls below the reference range (23 - 42). Do you see how the cortisol rhythm is "flattened" compared to normal? This person suffered from fatigue.

Free Cortisol Rhythm			
07:00 - 08:00 AM	22	Normal	13-24 nM
11:00 - Noon	3	Depressed	5-10 nM
04:00 - 05:00 PM	2	Depressed	3-8 nM
11:00 - Midnight	1	Normal	1-4 nM
Cortisol Burden:	28		23-42
DHEA	2	Depressed DHEA	Adults (M/F): 3-10
Dehydroepiandrosterone			

Figure -33.

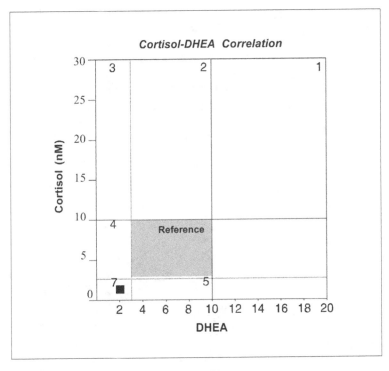

Figure -34.

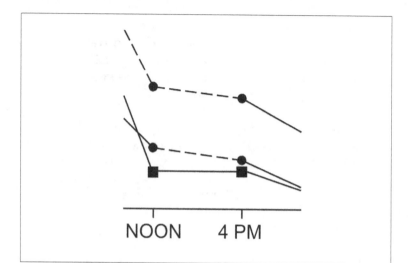

Figure -35.

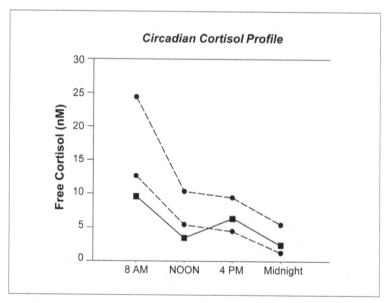

Figure -36.

* * *

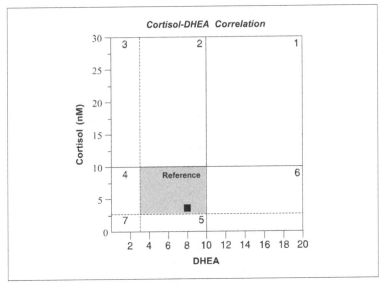

Figure -37.

Free Cortisol Rhythm

07:00 - 08:00 AM	9	Depressed	13-24 nM
11:00 - Noon	3	Depressed	5-10 nM
04:00 - 05:00 PM	5	Normal	3-8 nM
11:00 - Midnight	1	Normal	1-4 nM

Cortisol Burden:	19		23-42
DHEA	8	Normal	Adults (M/F): 3-10
Dehydroepiandrosterone			

Figure -38.

Here's another example of a person who suspected adrenal problems due to their symptoms. Their lab came back like this:

Again we see that the average of the Noon and 4 pm Cortisol amounts are within normal range, and the DHEA is OK.

But the total cortisol (Burden) is below normal.

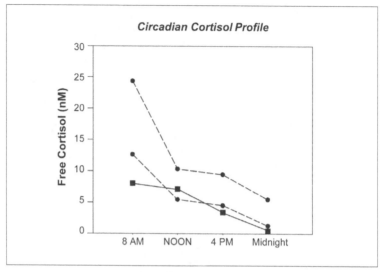

Figure -39.

Do you see where it says the final cortisol reading is < (less than) 0.3? If you search through Diagnostech.com and read through the technical articles, you will find this comment: Addison's Disease: < 1nM (any time)

The link to that quote cannot be done "directly" due to the way their site is set up; you have to click on "Tests & Panels" then "Conceptual Framework" then "Test Specifications". The same comment can be found on pg 36 of the 43 page Adrenal Stress Index manual provided to doctors, but I would not give anyone the label of "Addison's" until they had further testing done.

Nonetheless, it is noteworthy when there is immeasurable cortisol at any point of the day, as it certainly indicates that the person has low cortisol. And as the doctors have been quoted that the person lacks "adrenal reserve". They aren't coping with current cortisol needs, so how can they produce the extra cortisol needed during times of illness, or other stress such as bad news, car wreck, etc.?

It would be a mistake to simply glance at this person's reference zone and say it was a "Normal" result. You have to look at the cortisol rhythm, the total amount of cortisol they are making, and the symptoms of the patient that may are making, and the symptoms of the patient that may indicate adrenal fatigue (including blood pressure test upon standing, etc. (See Chapter 5.)

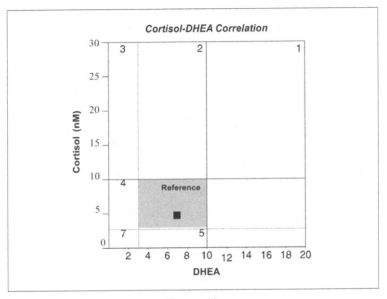

Figure -40.

Free Cortisol Rhythm			
07:00 - 08:00 AM	8	Depressed	13-24 nM
11:00 - Noon	7	Normal	5-10 nM
04:00 - 05:00 PM	2	Depressed	3-8 nM
11:00 - Midnight	<0.3		1-4 nM
Cortisol Burden:	17		23-42
DHEA	7	Normal	Adults (M/F): 3-10
Dehydroepiandrosterone			

Figure -41.

This lab result is kind of borderline.

As you can see, their cortisol burden is at the low end of normal, and the DHEA is below normal.

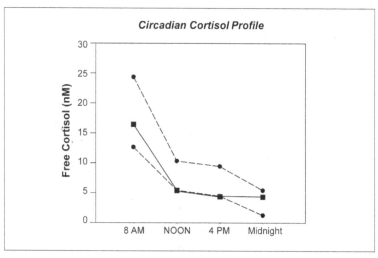

Figure - 42.

Free Cortisol Rhythm				_Freely in middle_
07:00 - 08:00 AM	16	Normal	13-24 nM	_18.5_
11:00 - Noon	5	Normal	5-10 nM	_7.5_
04:00 - 05:00 PM	3	Normal	3-8 nM	_5.5_
11:00 - Midnight	3	Normal	1-4 nM	_2.5_
				and borderline
Cortisol Burden:	27		23-42	_34_
DHEA Dehydroepiandrosterone	2	Depressed DHEA	Adults (M/F): 3-10	

Figure -43.

This person submitted a lab sample because she suspected adrenal fatigue due to her symptoms. This is an example where the DiagnosTechs Zone system is helpful. The mid-day cortisol amounts fall within the normal range (actually all her cortisol points are within normal). But the DHEA is low, and if you believe in the theory proposed by Dr. Selye, Dr. Peatfield, and others, this is an indicator that the adrenals are fatigued.

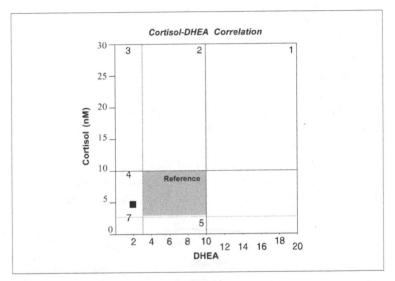

Figure -44.

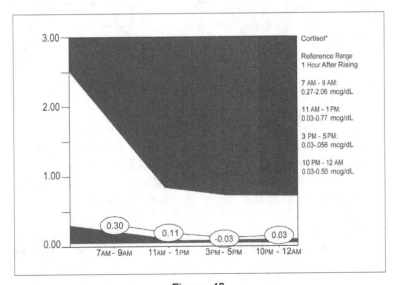

Figure -45.

So far, we have focused on the cortisol labs from Diagnos-Techs–but there are other labs that do these tests.

My doctor had boxes from Genova in his office so when I told him I wanted to get my adrenals checked he gave me their box.

I was fairly certain that I had adrenal fatigue. I had symptoms of chronic fatigue for 21 years following a severe viral illness (Epstein Barr).

Do you see how the Genova range of "normal" cortisol is hugging the bottom of the chart? It seems to go all the way down to "zero" on the cortisol measurement. I had immeasurable cortisol at 4 pm and it doesn't even appear out of range on the graph. My doctor had boxes from Genova in his office so when I told him I wanted to get my adrenals checked he gave me their box–it is at the edge of "normal".

There is no mention of cortisol burden. Genova labs show the DHEA like this. Mine was a bit lower than centerline.

Hormone	Reference Range		Reference Range
DHEA 7am - 9am	(120)		14-277 pg/mL
DHEA / Cortisol Ratio x 10,000		(400)	35-435

Figure - 46.

Now compare my labs, with immeasurable and barely measurable readings, to a woman's labs from DiagnosTechs, below. She has definite symptoms of adrenal fatigue over many years. After this lab test, her doctor gave her a prescription for Cortef.

As you can see, her cortisol burden "11" is about half of the low end of normal (23 - 42). Her lowest readings at any point of day are "2" and we have seen some DiagnosTechs examples at "1" and some that were not measurable (expressed as <

meaning "less than"). The way that DiagnosTechs charts the cortisol readings, it is very easy to compare with a "normal" range. When the result is low, you can evaluate HOW low.

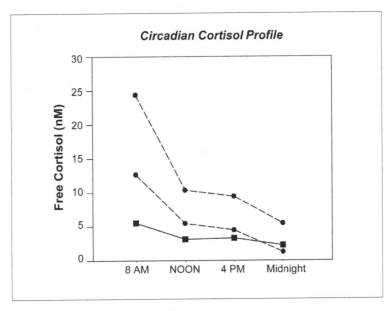

Figure -47.

Free Cortisol Rhythm			
07:00 - 08:00 AM	5	Depressed	13-24 nM
11:00 - Noon	2	Depressed	5-10 nM
04:00 - 05:00 PM	2	Depressed	3-8 nM
11:00 - Midnight	2	Normal	1-4 nM
Cortisol Burden:	11		23-42
DHEA Dehydroepiandrosterone	3	Borderline	Adults (M/F): 3-10

Figure -48.

I am of the personal opinion that the Genova lab range is overly broad, and that low levels of cortisol are hard to evaluate. I called them twice to discuss, left messages with whoever the receptionist transferred me to–and never got a call back.

This is a Cortisol-DHEA correlation. To me, this seems more useful than Genova's DHEA/Cortisol ratio. I can see at a glance if the Cortisol is high or low. I can see if the DHEA is high or low. The relationship of the 2 is clearly expressed.

* * *

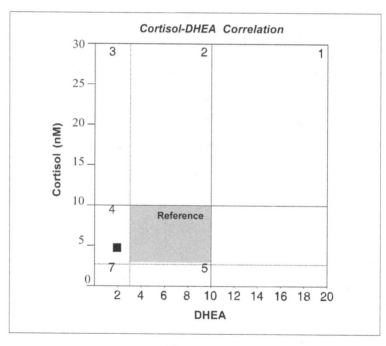

Figure -49.

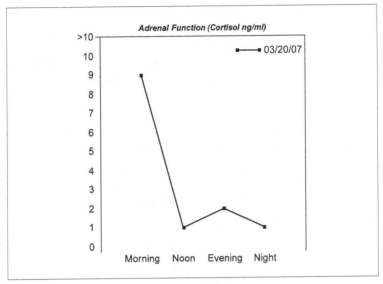

Figure -50.

Now let's look at an example from ZRT Labs

This member also gave permission to publish his chart (personal info removed) and described symptoms of adrenal fatigue. After receiving his lab result, he decided to treat his adrenals with Adrenal Cortex.

Hormone Test	In Range	Out Of Range	Units	Range
Estradiol (saliva)	1.0		pg/ml	0.8-2.2
Progesterone (saliva)	26		pg/ml	12-100
Testosterone (saliva)	80		pg/ml	44-148 (Age Dependent
DHEAS (saliva)	8.5		ng/ml	2-23 (Age Dependent)
Cortisol Morning (saliva)	9.0		ng/ml	3.7-9.5
Cortisol Noon (saliva)		1.1 L	ng/ml	1.2-3.0
Cortisol Evening (saliva)		2.2 H	ng/ml	0.6-1.9
Cortisol Night (saliva)	0.5		ng/ml	0.4-1.0
Free T4 (blood spot)	2.5		ng/dL	0.7-2.5
Free T3 (blood spot)		2.1 L	pg/ml	2.5-6.5
TSH (blood spot)	1.8		uU/ml	0.5-3.0
TPO (blood spot)		2247 H	IU/ml	0-150 (70-150 borderline)

Figure -51.

This person has an erratic rhythm–yet appears to have adequate cortisol production overall. I don't see ZRT commenting on the cortisol burden. One of the nice things about ZRT is they have the patient fill out a questionnaire and the report will comment on your symptoms as well as the measurement of cortisol.

IMPORTANT NOTE: There is a saliva test called Dutch, and sadly, we have often noted very wonky results, such as seeing high cortisol, but symptoms and results of other versions of saliva cortisol reveal the person actually has low cortisol. This strangeness doesn't happen all the time, but enough that it's important to mention.

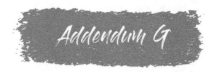

CONVERSION PATHWAYS

FROM CHOLESTEROL TO YOUR HORMONES

CHOLESTEROL
goes to
PREGNENOLONE
(with the help of thyroid hormones)

which then can go to
1) PROGESTERONE or 2) DHEA

1) PROGESTERONE can convert to
a) ALDOSTERONE, or...
b) CORTISOL, or...
c) ANDROSTENEDIONE, or...
d) TESTOSTERONE

2) DHEA will convert to
ANDROSTENEDIONE

ANDROSTENEDIONE
goes to
1) ESTROGENS and PROGESTERONE
(which can also come from the Ovaries)

or to

2) TESTOSTERONE
(which can also come from the Testes)

GLOSSARY

(WITH SOME HUMoR INCLUDED)

ACTH Stimulation (STIM):
Test which measures the level of cortisol before and after an injection of synthetic ACTH.

Adaptogens:
Any of several herbs used to help the body deal with stress and rejuvenate the adrenal glands. Works best with healthy adrenals under stress, not for those individuals who have proven low cortisol.

Addison's Disease:
Malfunction of the adrenal glands most commonly from an autoimmune destruction, causing an underproduction of cortisol

Adrenals:
Small glands which sit on top of each kidney and are chiefly responsible for our stress response, plus other important functions. They produce cortisol, adrenaline, aldosterone and DHEA, plus estrogen, progesterone, testosterone, and others.

Adrenal Dunce:
What patients will call their doctors when they pronounce that the only adrenal problems are Addison's and Cushing's

Adrenal Dysfunction:
Term to describe all problems with adrenals, which includes a mix of highs and lows, plus all lows. Sometimes includes low aldosterone.

Adrenal Fatigue:

Condition of sluggish adrenal function resulting in low cortisol levels, and sometimes low aldosterone. Excellent information on the last chapter of the Stop the Thyroid Madness II book.

Adrenal Insufficiency:

Condition of low cortisol production caused by Addison's disease, a progressive condition usually caused by an auto-immune attack. Thyroid patients will tend to get Adrenal Fatigue, not Adrenal Insufficiency.

Aldosterone:

Steroid produced by the adrenals, regulating sodium and potassium. You know it's low when it's midrange or lower, say years of experiences. Low aldosterone also causes most to pee more than they used to, or sweat more, or cause a desire for salty foods.

Armour:

Brand name of natural desiccated pig thyroid made by Forest Laboratories, Inc, a subsidiary of Allergen/ Activas

Antibodies:

Blood proteins produced by your immune system in response to a problem. Those with Hashimoto's will product antibodies against one's own thyroid.

Antidepressant:

A type of medication prescribed to treat depression.

Antithyroglobulin:

A Hashimoto's antibody directed against the protein thyroglobulin, which is important for thyroid hormone production.

Autoimmune:

Refers to an immune system going haywire, attacking its

own cells and tissues, such as Celiac, Hashimoto's, Diabetes Type 1, Lupus, Rheumatoid Arthritis, etc. See the book *Hashimoto's: Taming the Beast*

B12:
Vitamin which maintains healthy nerves and red blood cells. Optimal puts it in the upper quarter of a range. If too low, or not being broken down for us, patients report noticed their fingers, hands or legs going asleep too fast.

Butthead:
How patients have internally described their doctors when the doctor pooh-poohed their continuing hypothyroid symptoms while on a T4-only med.

Carbohydrates:
Organic compounds in foods that supply energy and include simple sugars like glucose or complex sugars like cellulose or starch.

Calcitonin:
Hormone produced by the thyroid which helps prevent too-high levels of calcium in your serum, and in turn improves bone strength. Found in desiccated thyroid.

CFS:
Abbreviation for Chronic Fatigue Syndrome, a condition that many feel is untreated or undertreated hypothyroid.

Corticosteroid:
Class of adrenal steroid hormone which is anti-inflammatory, like cortisol.

Cortisol:
A corticosteroid hormone produced by the adrenals, also called the stress hormone; In healthy individuals, it's highest in the early morning, lowest at bedtime.

Cushing's Syndrome:
Disease of the adrenals causing over-production of cortisol.

Cytomel (liothyronine sodium):
Brand name for synthetic T3

DHEA:
Hormone secreted by the adrenal glands which is a precursor to testosterone. It falls every decade of our life.

Deiodinases (or 5' deiodinases):
Enzymes from peripheral tissues, and mostly the liver, which help conversion of T4 to T3 by taking off an iodine atom from the outer ring of T4. RT3 is made when an iodine atom is removed from inner ring. These enzymes can be faulty because of mutations.

D.O.
Abbreviation for Doctor of Osteopathy. Osteopathy is based on the idea of treating the whole person.

Desiccated Thyroid:
Term for prescription porcine pig thyroid that has been dried and powdered, containing exactly what the human thyroid makes–T4, T3, T2, T1 and calcitonin. Can also be bovine in over the counter versions.

Electric Shock Therapy (EST):
A treatment of voltage thought to decrease depression. Janie Bowthorpe's mother was sadly put through this procedure instead of the doctor figuring out that her depression was due to Synthroid.

Eltroxin:
Brand name of synthetic T4 (levothyroxine, thyroxine) medication.

Endocrine glands:
Glands that secrete hormones into the blood, including the pituitary gland, pancreas, gonads, thyroid and adrenals.

Endocrinologist:
A doctor who specializes in the Endocrine System. Patients complain the most about the rigidity of Endos and their obsession with T4-only medications and the TSH. There can be rare exceptions.

Estrogen:
Steroid acting mainly as a female hormone, and occurs as either estradiol, estriol and estrone.

Estrogen dominance:
Condition where the female hormone estrogen is too high as compared to progesterone levels, and unopposed. Some mutations cause estrogen not to be broken down well.

Euthyroidism:
Being normal in thyroid function. Some doctors will unfortunately use the phrase simply because of a normal TSH.

Ferritin:
Iron storage protein. If it goes high, that points to inflammation, as the body will push iron into storage with inflammation.

Fibromyalgia:
A condition characterized by widespread pain in the muscles and joints, and includes fatigue, sleep disorders, and depression. The pain associated with a poor thyroid treatment can be diagnosed as fibromyalgia.

Florinef (fludrocortisone acetate):
Prescription corticosteroid drug with some glucocorticoid potency, but with greater mineralcorticoid potency, used for

low aldosterone levels.

Free Thyroxine Index (FTI or F7):
Tells how much T4 is present compared to the thyroxine-binding globulin; Is considered an outdated lab test.

Garbage can:
Where many thyroid patients have thrown their T4 medications after they got on desiccated thyroid and lived again.

Glucocorticoid:
A steroid adrenal hormone of which the most abundant is cortisol.

Glycyrrhizin acid:
Molecule found in the licorice plant which extends the life of cortisol by inhibiting enzyme responsible for inactivating cortisol in the kidneys.

Goiter:
Enlargement of the thyroid gland.

Grave's Disease:
Hyperthyroidism, or overactivity of the thyroid gland. Usually due to an autoimmune process.

Hashimoto's Disease:
An autoimmune attack on the thyroid gland which can result in inflammation and causes swings between hyperthyroid and hypothyroid. See the book **Hashimoto's: Taming the Beast**

Hepatitis:
A blood-borne virus which affects the liver negatively; often caused by intravenous or nasal drug use, tattoos or unsafe sex or social practices.

Hoodwinked:
How thyroid patients feel when they find out that all the antidepressants, cholesterol meds and other medications may not have been needed if they had been on desiccated thyroid and optimal. T4/T3 can do the same.

Hydrocortisone (HC):
Prescription synthetic cortisol medication, often used when saliva cortisol is quite low.

Hyperthyroidism:
Condition of excess thyroid function and hormones. Sometimes is used wrong to describe the symptoms of excess adrenaline due to low cortisol.

Hypopituitary:
Sluggish or damaged pituitary gland negatively affecting the release of messenger hormones like the TSH, ACTH, growth hormone, etc.

Hypothalamus:
Small gland in the brain which sends messages to the pituitary to release messenger hormones to stimulate the adrenals and thyroid.

Hypothyroidism:
Condition of insufficient thyroid function and hormones. Can be caused by autoimmune Hashimoto's, non-Hashi's hypothyroidism, removal of thyroid gland, etc.

Insulin:
Hormone from the pancreas that enables cells to take in blood sugar (glucose).

Iodine:
Naturally-occurring element which is key to good health, and of which thyroid hormones are primarily composed. Supplemental iodine is either Lugol's (liquid) or Iodoral

(tablets). There are other brands and versions.

Iodine Loading Test:
Urine test used to determine if iodine levels are sufficient.

L-Thyroxine:
Another name for T4, the storage thyroid hormone. Same as just thyroxine.

Levothyroxine:
Generic term for all synthetic T4-only medications.

Levoxyl:
Brand name of a synthetic T4-only medication by King Pharmaceuticals.

Liothyronine:
Generic term for synthetic T3-only medications.

Lithium:
Prescription drug used to treat bipolar disorder, and which also inhibits thyroid function.

Medrol (Methylprednisolone):
A synthetic cortisol prescription medication used to treat inflammation and improve symptoms of certain disorders.

Melatonin:
A hormone which regulates our circadian rhythm to cause drowsiness.

Metabolism:
Chemical reactions which give energy. Great improved with T3 in one's treatment, which desiccated thyroid also gives.

Mineralcorticoid:
Class of adrenal steroid hormone which promotes sodium retention and fluid balance, like aldosterone.

Mitral Valve Prolapse (MVP):
A mostly benign condition of the heart resulting in a floppy mitral valve and slight regurgitation. Janie Bowthorpe has this.

Moron:
How a thyroid patient describes his or her doctor after the doc says desiccated thyroid is outdated or the TSH is the best test.

Myxedema:
Skin and tissue thickening and puffiness caused by hypothyroidism.

Natural Desiccated Thyroid:
Another name for desiccated thyroid.

Naturethroid:
A brand of natural desiccated pig thyroid by RLC Labs, formerly Western Research Labs.

Naturopathy:
An alternative form of medicine with a holistic approach and which may include homeopathy, herbs, acupuncture, aromatherapy, and others.

Nimcompoop:
What a patient called her doctor when he thought it was okay to hold her on one grain of desiccated thyroid for six weeks before raising.

Nodule:
A small and abnormal lump on the thyroid, mostly benign with 10% being cancerous.

NP Thyroid:
Brand name of natural desiccated thyroid by Acella Labs.

Nutri-Meds:
Brand name of non-prescription form of desiccated thyroid, bovine or porcine.

Oroxine:
Australian brand of synthetic T4, as is Eutroxsig.

Osteopathy:
Medical approach that emphasizes the role of the musculoskeletal system in health or disease.

Osteopenia:
Having weaker bones and often a precursor to having Osteoporosis. Many report it being reversed once they got on desiccated thyroid and became optimal.

Osteoporosis:
A calcium-wasting bone disease making bones brittle and easily broken. Some patients on T4-only see this happen to them.

Pale:
The color a patient's face turns when doc says the TSH is too low while on desiccated thyroid or T3. (false)

Palpitation:
An abnormal heartbeat; sudden extra-beat. Can occur with a cortisol problem when raising NDT or T3. Also common to having Mitral Valve Prolapse.

Percent Saturation:
Lab test which measures the percentage of iron bound to and carried around by the protein transferrin. It can be obtained by the serum iron divided by TIBC. Optimal for women is ~35; for men, ~38.

Pituitary Gland:
Small gland in the base of the brain which sends stimulating messengers to other glands, including the thyroid and adrenals. The TSH is one of those messenger hormones.

Phosphatidylserine (PS):
A nutrient of which half is in our brain cells; the supplement is said to boost brain power, plus lower high cortisol levels.

Potassium:
An essential mineral found in many foods and chemically similar to sodium, but balances sodium levels.

Pregnenolone:
Steroid hormone, also called the prohormone that converts down to other hormones.

Primary Adrenal Fatigue:
Sluggish adrenal function resulting in low cortisol and found as a poor function in the adrenals themselves like Addison's disease.

Progesterone:
Steroid hormone involved in menstruation and pregnancy. Can convert to cortisol.

RAI (Radioactive Iodine):
The use of radioactive iodine in the treatment of hyperthyroidism which slows down the activity of the thyroid. Considered unnecessary and with too many potential side effects by a growing body of thyroid patients in favor of blocking medications.

Renin:
An enzyme released from the kidneys in response to decreased salt levels. Helps regulate one's blood pressure.

Reverse T3:

The inactive form of T3 made by T4 conversion; Made when the body needs to decrease its T4. In thyroid patients, can go high due to low iron, inflammation, and high cortisol.

Stop the Thyroid Madness:

A term coined by author, blogger, coach, and website creator Janie Bowthorpe to describe a patient revolution for better thyroid treatment.

Secondary Adrenal Fatigue:

Sluggish adrenal function caused by Hypopituitary, or the failure to send the ACTH messenger to stimulate the adrenals

Selenium:

A trace mineral important for good health and which promotes the conversion of T4 to T3. Selenium also lowers anti-TPO Hashimoto's antibodies. Literature states 200-400 mcg is safe.

Serum iron:

The small amount of circulating iron which is bound by the protein transferrin.

Stupidly:

The way the TSH lab test discovers hypothyroid i.e. it takes years to rise high enough while we are hypothyroid.

Synthroid:

Form of synthetic T4 made by Abbott Laboratories.

Subclinical hypothyroidism:

Term for a supposed mild form of hypothyroid, though it's often the diagnosis of a doctor who relies solely on a TSH lab result rather than clear symptoms.

T3:

Active form of thyroid hormone, also called triiodothyronine.

T4:
Storage form of thyroid hormone

T4-only:
Shortened name for a thyroxine-only medication like Synthroid, Levoxy, Eltoxin, Oroxine, etc.

Testosterone:
Steroid hormone secreted in the testes of males and the ovaries of females.

Testy:
How a patient gets if one more doctor proclaims she or he is "normal".

Thyroid:
Butterfly shaped gland which has a major role in our energy levels and good health.

Thyroid Hormone Resistance:
Syndrome of poor cellular response to thyroid hormones, causing a patient to need higher doses to get the same effect of lower doses. Is genetic.

Thyroid Peroxidase (TPOab):
Enzyme that is important in the formation of the thyroid hormone. Often attacked with Hashimoto's disease. See the book Hashimoto's: Taming the Beast

Thyroiditis:
An umbrella term that includes Hashimoto's or inflammation of the thyroid.

Thyrotropin Releasing Hormone (TRH):
Hormone released by the Hypothalamus to send a message to the Pituitary gland, so that the latter will release other messenger hormones like the TSH.

Thyroxine:
Name for T4, the thyroid storage hormone.

Thyroxine-binding globulin test:
Measures the level of thyroid hormone-binding proteins.

TIBC:
Stands for Total Iron Binding Capacity and measures the ability of the transferrin protein to do its job in carrying iron to your liver, bone marrow and spleen. Will go high when iron is low, or high when iron is high due to the MTHFR gene or other methylation cause.

Triiodothyronine:
Name for T3, the active thyroid hormone.

TSH:
Thyroid Stimulating Hormone, secreted by the pituitary to stimulate the thyroid to produce/release thyroid hormones. The test and it's ridiculous normal range constantly fails us.

Unithroid:
Brand name of synthetic T4 made by Jerome Stevens Pharmaceuticals.

Wilson's Syndrome:
Condition   of high levels of Reverse T3 and low body temperature, coined by an MD of the same name. More for those without true hypothyroidism, but having RT3 due to stress. Treatment has harmed some true hypothyroid patients, they state.

WP Thyroid:
Brand of natural desiccated thyroid hormone by RLC Labs,

REFERENCES

Sometimes URL's go to now-defunct websites, or the page name changes on the existing website. If that happens, just do a search for the subject or title.

Academy of Osteopaths:
http://www.academyofosteopathy.org

Acella Pharmaceuticals, LLC
https://www.acellapharma.com/

Adrenal Fatigue: *http://adrenalfatigue.org/*

Alevizaki, Maria, Emily Mantzou, Adriana T. Cimponeriu, Calliope C. Alevizaki and Dimitri A. Koutras: TSH may not be a good marker for adequate thyroid hormone replacement therapy. 20 June 2005, Website: *www. springerlink. com/ content/y28n557300582h33/*

American College for the Advancement of Medicine: Doctors Armour. Website: *www.acam.org/dr_search/index.php*

Arem, Ridha, M.D. The Thyroid Solution: A Mind Body Program for Beating Depression and Regaining Your Emotional and Physical Health. New York: Ballantine Books, 2000

Barnes, Broda O., M.D., & Lawrence Galton: Hypothyroidism: the Unsuspected Illness. New York: Harper & Row, 1976 Website: *www.BrodaBarnes.org*

Chatzipanagiotou, S, J.N. Legakis, F. Boufidou, V. Petroyianm, C. Nicolaou: Prevalence of Yersini plasmid-encoded outer protein (Yop) class-specific antibodies in patients with Hashimoto's thyroiditis. 2001 Website: *www. blackwell-synergy.com/doi/pdf/10.1046/j.1469-*

0691.2001.00221.x?cookieSet=1

Brownstein, David, M.D. Overcoming Thyroid Disorders: WestBloomfield, MI. Medical Alternatives Press. 2002

National Celiac: Website: *www.csaceliacs.org/*

Cytomel Product Information: *https://www.pfizer.com/products/product-detail/cytomel*

Derry, David M.D: Email to Janie Bowthorpe 2006

Derry, David, MD, Ph.D.: Breast Cancer and Iodine: How to Prevent and How to Survive Breast Cancer. Trafford Publishing, 2001

DiagnosTechs, Inc: *www.diagnostechs.com/main.htm*

Direct Laboratory Services, Inc: Website: *www.directlabs.com/*

Durrant-Peatfield, Barry, M.B., B.S., LR.C.P., M.RCS: The Great Thyroid Scandal and How to Survive It. London, UK Barons Down Publishing, 2002.

Durrant-Peatfield, Barry, M.B., B.S., LR.C.P., M.RCS: Your Thyroid and How to Keep It Healthy. London, UK, Hammersmith Press Limited; 2Rev Ed edition

Encyclopedia Britannica: George Redmayne Murray Website: *www.britannica.com/eb/article-9054362/George-Redmayne-Murray*

Endocrine Web: Website: *www.endocrineweb.com/hypo1.html*

Erfa Canadian Thyroid.
www.erfa-sa.com/thyroid_en.htm

Genova Diagnostics: Website: *www.gdx.net/home/*

Goodman, Louis S., and Alfred Gilman: The Pharmacological Basis of Therapeutics. Toronto: The MacMillan Company,

Heinrich, Thomas, W, MD, Garth Graham, MD: Hypothyroidism Presented as Psychosis: Myxedema Madness Revisited. Primary Care Companion Journal of Clinical *References 261* Psychiatry 2003:5. Website: *www.psychiatrist.com/pcc/pccpdf/v05n06/v05n0603.pdf*

Holmes, Diana Tears Behind Closed Doors, 2nd edition: Wolverhampton, UK: Normandi Publishing Ltd, 2002

Honeyman-Lowe, Gina, and John C. Lowe: Your Guide to Metabolic Health. Lafayette, CO: McDowell Health-Science Books, 2003

Jorde, R., J. Sundsfjord. Serum TSH Levels in Smokers and Non-Smokers: The 5th Tromsø Study. Exp Clin Endocrinol Diabetes 2006; 114: 343-347 DOI: 10.1055/s-2006-924264. Website: *www.thieme-connect.com/ejournals/abstract/eced/doi/10.1055/s-2006-924264*

Kendall, Edward C. Journal of Biological Chemistry:

Lam, Michael, MD. Website: *www.drlam.com/A3R_brief_in_doc_format/adrenal_fatigue.cfm*

Lowe, John D., DC. Addenda to: Four 2003 Studies of Thyroid Hormone Replacement Therapies: Logical Analysis and Ethical Implications, 2003.Website: *www.drlowe.com/frf/t4replacement/addenda.htm*

Natural Thyroid Hormone Users Yahoo Group, started by Janie Bowthorpe in 2002: Website: *http://health.groups.yahoo. com/group/NaturalThyroidHormones*

Nobel Prize Information: Website: *http://nobelprize.org/*

Northrup, Christiane, MD: Website: *www.drnorthrup.com/*

NPTech Clinical Laboratory: Website: *www.pathlab.com.au/*

Rack, SK and EH Makela: Hypothyroidism and depression: a therapeutic challenge. The Annals of Pharmacotherapy: Vol. 34, No. 10, pp. 1142-1145, 2000 Harvey Whitney Books Company. Website: *www.theannals.com/cgi/content/abstract/34/10/1142*

Swartout, Hubert O., MD, DNB, Ph.D.: Modern Medical Counselor, Washington, DC Review and Herald Publishing Association 1951

Rind, David, MD: Website: *www.drrind.com*

Rousset, Bernard A. Ph.D., John T. Dunn, M.D: Thyroid Hormone Synthesis and Secretion, Chapter 2, *www. thyroidmanager.org/Chapter2/2-frame.htm, 13 April 2004*

Shomon, Mary, David M. Derry M.D., Ph.D: Rethinking the TSH Test: An Interview with David Derry, M.D., Ph.D., *www.thyroid-info.com/articles/david-derry.htm*

Simoni, Robert D., Robert L. Hill, and Martha Vaughan. The Isolation of Thyroxine and Cortisone: the Work of Edward C. Kendall. J. Biol. Chem., Vol. 277, Issue 21, 10, May 24, 2002

Sriprasit Pharma Co. Ltd: *www.sriprasit.com/en/us/index. asp*

United States Pharmacopeia: Website: *www.usp.org/ aboutUSP/*

Unithroid Product Information: Website: *www.unithroid.com*

Westhroid Product Information: Website: *www.rlclabs.com*

Wilson, James L. ND. Adrenal Fatigue, The 21st Century Stress Syndrome: Petaluma, CA. Smart Publications; 1st edition, 2002

Ybarra, T. R. Britons Discover Synthetic Thyroxin: New York Times, Dec. 12, 1927

RESOURCES

Though this Stop the Thyroid Madness book is a unique in its focus as a patient-to-patient book, there are other resources that might be of interest. This is not an exhaustive list of good books.

SUPPLEMENTAL READING:

Hashimoto's: Taming the Beast
By Janie A. Bowthorpe M.Ed.

Collecting years of Hashimoto's patient experiences, this compilation teaches the reader about autoimmunity, stages of Hashi's, environmental and genetic triggers, gut health issues (two chapters!), foods and supplements, and more importantly, how Hashimoto's patients have reported getting well. It's purposely concise and to the point so there aren't excess pages to get through! *laughinggrapepublishing.com*

Your Thyroid and How to Keep it Healthy
by Dr. Barry Durrant-Peatfield, MB BS LRCP MRCS

Though we went beyond this book in the adrenal arena as shown in this book's chapters 5 and 6, it's his Second Edition of *The Great Thyroid Scandal and How to Survive It*, and it is filled with excellent information about the thyroid, hypo- and hyper, iodine, female hormones and testosterone, plus adrenals.

Safe Uses of Cortisol
by William McK. Jefferies, M.D., F. A. C. P.

This was our learning manual at the beginning about adrenals and cortisol use. It includes therapeutic recommendations and important aspects of cortisone or cortisol in patients with chronic allergies, autoimmune disorders, and chronic fatigue. Incredible gems of information.

Pets at Risk: From Allergies to Cancer, Remedies for an unsuspected Epidemic by Alfred J. Plechner DVM & Martin Zucker

Yes, believe it or not, this veterinarian's book about pets has some gems of information about adrenals that can apply to humans. Plechner describes a problem in the endocrine and immune system, including the adrenals, that causes a lot of problems that involves treatment with pharmaceutical meds as well as diet.

The Paleo Thyroid Solution by Elle Russ

This book provides the only lifestyle and weight loss plan specifically targeted for maximizing thyroid hormone metabolism in harmony with paleo/primal/ancestral health principles.

Adrenal Fatigue: The 21st-Century Stress Syndrome by James L. Wilson, N.D., D.C., Ph.D.

Though this will not go into the patient-to-patient details in this book's chapters 5 and 6, it's still a friendly, easy-to-read book about adrenal issues which are common with hypothyroid patients. The book opens with an overview of the function of the adrenals, and how they are prone to chronic fatigue given our hyper-stressed contemporary lifestyles. It continues with information on how to tell if you have adrenal fatigue and multiple strategies for treatment.

Why Do I Still have Thyroid Symptoms When my Lab Tests are Normal by Datis Kharrazian

This book contains unique information about the *Th1 and Th2* inflammation cytokines and how to find out which you lean towards with Hashimoto's. Kharrazian outlines his successes in balancing the immune system.

Your Guide to Metabolic Health, co-authored by Dr. Gina Honeyman, DC and Dr. John Lowe, DC.

This informative book outlines poor metabolic health, which

includes low energy, aches and pains, depression, poor memory and concentration, anxiety, malaise, etc., and moves into good information on the two most common causes– untreated or under-treated hypothyroidism and thyroid hormone resistance.

Hormones, Health, and Happiness: A Natural Medical Formula for Rediscovering Youth
by Steven F. Hotze, M.D.

In an 8-point program, Hotze describes a new model of healthcare, using bio-identical hormones and other natural treatments. It goes against the prevailing medical approach of treating individual symptoms with the familiar "anti" drugs– such as antibiotics, antihistamines, and antidepressants, and instead addresses the underlying causes of poor health.

Hypothyroidism: The Unsuspected Illness
by Broda O. Barnes, M.D. and Lawrence Galton

A classic from 1976, this easy-to-read and pioneering book explains the thyroid gland, how it works, and problems its dysfunction can induce. Includes detailed case histories of patients, often who were thought hopeless, whose problems were discovered to be related to hypothyroidism and were cured by Dr. Barnes' simple effective techniques, included basal temperature taking and the use of desiccated thyroid.

Hypothyroidism Type 2: The Epidemic
by Mark Starr, M.D.

A clear and understandable explanation of why so many people today are suffering from hypothyroidism, despite "normal" blood tests. Has information on the cause and successful treatment for obesity, heart attacks, depression, diabetes, strokes, headaches, chronic fatigue, and others. In Dr. Starr's description, he presents overwhelming evidence showing a majority of Americans suffer this illness, which is due to environmental and hereditary factors.

The Great Thyroid Scandal and How To Survive It by
Dr. Barry Durrant-Peatfield, MB, BS, LRCP, MRCS
  An excellent review of thyroid disease and the treatment
alternatives using natural glandular extracts (desiccated
thyroid) and adrenal support like cortisol. The book takes you
step by step through the diagnosis and treatment of thyroid
illnesses and reveals how poorly modern medicine understands
thyroid disease.

Overcoming Thyroid Disorders by Dr. David Brownstein
  This book is holistically oriented in the treatment of
hypothyroidism, and shows how a natural treatment program
consisting of natural thyroid hormone, other natural hormones,
vitamins, minerals, diet modifications and detoxification can
successfully treat many conditions. It includes over 30 actual
cases from his practice. A hopeful book.

*The Hormone Solution: Stay Younger Longer with
Natural Hormone and Nutrition Therapies*
by Thierry Dr. Hertoghe MD
  This book presents an effective program to counter memory
loss, weight gain, poor muscle mass, hair loss and many
other symptoms of aging. He recommends the use of natural
hormones along with a healthy diet plus supplementation of
certain minerals and vitamins. He outlines the 15 main and
crucial hormones found in your body and how each helps
restore the others.

*The Thyroid Solution: A Mind-Body Program for
Beating Depression and Regaining Your Emotional
and Physical Health* by Arem Ridha, M.D.
  Examines the fundamentals of thyroid disease, including
diagnosis and therapy, although the focus is on the significance
of the thyroid in cognition and emotions. It explains the link
between stress and thyroid imbalance; how thyroid imbalance
affects your emotions, sex life, and relationships; and how to
cope with the effects of this imbalance. A whole section deals
with women's health issues.

Thyroid - Guardian of Health by Philip G. Young, M.D.

This overall reference book examines the impact inadequate thyroid function has on individuals and the fact that hypothyroidism is frequently missed. Include history, environmental factor, and frequent clinical presentations of hypothyroidism, blood tests and their faults. Thyroid's relationship to adrenal hormones is also discussed

Tears Behind Closed Doors by Diana Holmes

This book is an examination of a serious medical problem (untreated/undertreated hypothyroidism) and is the result of the author's untiring crusade to prevent others from going through the physical and emotional hell she had to endure. It is a positive personal account that will give comfort and inspiration.

Salt: Your Way to Health by David Brownstein, MD

Dr. Brownstein not only debunks the low-salt diet / lowered blood pressure myth, he gives you clear and concise reasons for adding unrefined salt to one's daily regimen. He shows you how an adequate salt intake is necessary for proper functioning of the hormonal system and the immune system and that includes proper adrenal function.

Could It Be B12?: An Epidemic of Misdiagnoses
by Sally M. Pacholok RN and Jeffrey J. Stuart DO

A silent crippler stalks millions of Americans and you maybe one of them... is how this excellent book starts out about the common problem of a B12 deficiency. The book describes the different manifestations of low B12; including the fact that it can mimic MS or other neurological disorders, as well as cause mental illness, learning disabilities, impaired immune function, plus more. A must read for those who suspect they have low B12.

The Metabolic Treatment of Fibromyalgia
by John C. Lowe
This acclaimed book is equal to a very large textbook and chock full of excellent medical information and research, revealing what a very intelligent and meticulous man Lowe was. He goes into great detail explaining the treatment, how well patients respond to a combination of T4 and T3, and even with a "normal" lab result. He mentions important dietary practices in the treatment.

WEBSITES

http://stopthethyroidmadness.com/ Patient-to-patient website compiled by Janie Bowthorpe, M.Ed.

https://tinyurl.com/saliva-cortisol An excellent saliva test you can order yourself

http://www.drplechner.com/ Brilliant website about the adrenal status and treatment of animals by Dr. Alfred Plechner that could aptly be compared to humans!

www.drrind.com One of our favorite sites for a downloadable graph and instructions for temperature-taking–a must!

www.thyroidmanager.org Where you can find the reference that the thyroid produces an equivalence of 3-5 grains, and more!

www.naturalthyroidchoices.com Not copyright updated, but still contains good info by Stephanie, who won her battle with thyroid cancer, plus information on children and thyroid.

www.breastcancerchoices.org/ This website shows a strong connection between the use of iodine (which also benefits your thyroid) and breast health.

www.drginahoneyman.com Website of Dr. Honeyman, who heads the Center for Metabolic Health and who co-authored a Metabolic book with Lowe.

www.earthclinic.com I LOVE this site. Filled with patient information on treatment that worked on various ills.

www.theguthealthprotocol.com For Hashimoto's patients in dealing with their gut issues

Patient-to-patient groups

http://stopthethyroidmadness.com/talk-to-others

T-shirts, bumper stickers, business cards, baby items and so much more to spread the word!!

http://stopthethyroidmadness.com/t-shirt

INDEX

I

Has this book changed your life?

Found information here that you can find nowhere else?

Want others to have this information?

Please visit the publisher's website at:

www.laughinggrapepublishing.com/

to order more copies of this book for friends or relatives.

For t-shirts, bumperstickers, clothing, baby clothes, magnets, and more to spread the word to others. : *www.stopthethyroidmadness.com/t-shirt*

You're not very good at listening to instructions, are you? :)

But that actually means you can be your own best advocate instead of blindly following bad information! Seize the wisdom of thyroid patients before you!

Janie A. Bowthorpe. M.Ed.